Children with Special Health Care and Nutritional Needs

Behavioral Health Nutrition Dietetic Practice
Group and Pediatric Nutrition Practice Group

Edited by Jacque DeVore, MPH, RD,
and Andrea Shotton, MS, RD

eat right. Academy of Nutrition
and Dietetics

Diana Faulhaber, Publisher
Krisan Matthews, Development Editor
Elizabeth Nishiura, Production Manager

10 9 8 7 6 5 4 3 2 1

Contents

Contributors

EDITORS

Jacque Devore, MPH, RD
Shriners Hospital for Children Portland
Portland, OR

Andrea Shotton, MS, RD
Therapy Works, Inc
Tulsa, OK

AUTHORS

Marion Taylor Baer, PhD, RD
USC Keck School of Medicine
USC University Center for Excellence in Developmental
    Disabilities (UCEDD)
Children's Hospital Los Angeles
Los Angeles, CA

Liz Enagonio, MS, RD, CNSC
Kennedy Krieger Institute
Baltimore, MD

Cary B. Kreutzer, MPH, RD
USC University Center for Excellence in Developmental
    Disabilities (UCEDD)
Children's Hospital Los Angeles
Los Angeles, CA

Jackie Krick, MS, RD
Kennedy Krieger Institute
Baltimore, MD

Mildred K. Leatham, MPH, RD, CHES
USC University Center for Excellence in Developmental
    Disabilities (UCEDD)
Children's Hospital Los Angeles
Los Angeles, CA

Patricia Miller, MS, RD, CSP
Kennedy Krieger Institute
Baltimore, MD

Patricia Murray, MEd, RD
New Hampshire Department of Health and Human
    Services
Special Medical Services
Concord, NH

Aaron Owens, MS, RD, CSP, CD
Seattle Children's Hospital
Seattle, WA

Sharon C. Weston, MS, RD
Children's Hospital Boston
Boston, MA

Janet H. Willis, MPH, RD
Virginia LEND Program
Richmond, VA

L. Hope Wills, MA, RD, CSP, CLS
USC University Center for Excellence in Developmental
    Disabilities (UCEDD)
Children's Hospital Los Angeles
Los Angeles, CA

Reviewers

Monica Cohen, RD
Alfred I. Dupont Hospital for Children
Palmyra, NJ

Marisa A. Dzarnoski, RD
The Children's Hospital
Aurora, CO

Michelle L. Henry, MPH, RD
The Children's Hospital
Aurora, CO

Janice M. Vickerstaff Joneja, PhD, RD
Vickerstaff Health Services, Inc.
Kamloops, BC, Canada

Susan Konek, MA, RD, CSP
The Children's Hospital of Philadelphia
Philadelphia, PA

Paula Charuhas Macris, MS, RD, CSO, FADA, CD
Seattle Cancer Care Alliance
Seattle, WA

Esther F. Myers, PhD, RD, FADA
Academy of Nutrition and Dietetics
Chicago, IL

Patricia Novak, MPH, RD, CLE
Pasadena Child Development Associates
Sherman Oaks, CA

Lee Shelly Wallace, MS, RD, FADA
Boling Center for Developmental Disabilities
University of Tennessee Health Science Center
Memphis, TN

Wendy Wittenbrook, MA, RD, CSP
Texas Scottish Rite Hospital for Children
Dallas, TX

Acknowledgments

As with many books published by the Academy of Nutrition and Dietetics, the creation of this pocket guide would not have been accomplished if it were not for a team of exceptional professionals. We would like to acknowledge the efforts of the authors, reviewers, and Academy staff members who aided the development of this publication. Executive committees of both the Behavioral Health Nutrition (BHN) and Pediatric Nutrition Practice Group (PNPG) dietetic practice groups also supported the publication of the pocket guide. If not for their recognition of the importance of updating practice guidelines based upon new scientific evidence, the guide would not have been completed. Academy staff members Krisan Matthews and Nancy Barbour provided the much needed guidance and expertise in all technical aspects of producing a "pocket-sized" guide. We wish to thank them for their ongoing assistance and support.

Most significantly, we would like to thank our families for their overwhelming support and understanding of the time constraints in each phase of development of the publication.

Jacque DeVore, MPH, RD
Andrea Shotton, MS, RD

Foreword

The *Academy of Nutrition and Dietetics Pocket Guide to Children with Special Health Care and Nutritional Needs* is a valuable quick-reference tool for health care professionals serving this population, whether in clinical settings, management, or community dietetics. This pocket guide represents the collaborative efforts of the Behavioral Health Nutrition Dietetic Practice Group (DPG) and the Pediatric Nutrition Practice Group, and it presents the most up-to-date, interdisciplinary research- and evidence-based information available on the nutrition management of children with special health care needs (CSHCN). The book is a must-have for everyone who serves the CSHCN population throughout the community.

The Behavioral Health Nutrition DPG is proud to have past chair, Andrea Shotton, MS, RD, serve as coeditor of this pocket guide. Her coeditor, Jacque De Vore, MPH, RD, from the Pediatric Nutrition DPG, brings 25 years of experience working with the pediatric special needs population in both public health and hospital settings to this project. We want to congratulate Andrea and Jacque on their efforts in putting this pocket guide together. We hope this up-to-date information will help health care providers who are interested in this essential area of practice and those who provide critical support to these children with varied nutritional needs.

Charlotte Caperton-Kilburn, MS, RD, CSSD
Chair, Behavioral Health Nutrition DPG, 2011–2012

Beverly W. Henry, PhD, RD
Chair, Pediatric Nutrition Practice Group, 2010–2011

Introduction

The term *children with special health care needs* (CSHCN) refers to children with a broad range of chronic illnesses and conditions who require health and related services beyond basic, routine care. Intervention generally includes a range of medical, therapy, educational, financial, and family support services. CSHCN includes children with birth defects, neurological consequences of premature birth, genetic syndromes, sequelae of infection such as meningitis, and consequences of perinatal drug exposure. Also included in the definition of CSHCN are those "at risk" for chronic physical, developmental, and behavior conditions, such as children with very low birth weight, metabolic disorders, extreme poverty, or environmental exposures, such as exposure to secondhand smoke or lead.

In many ways, children with special health care needs are similar to children without special health care needs. All children require good nutrition to grow and develop. As a group, however, CSHCN have more frequent problems that may alter their growth, diet, feeding and eating behaviors, and bowel and fluid management. When these problems are not adequately addressed, a child may experience more infections and illness and spend fewer days in school or therapy, while health care costs for the family increase. These feeding and nutrition-related problems are also more likely to be chronic over time. The following are the most common challenges:

- Altered growth (eg, underweight, overweight, or short stature)
- Inadequate energy and nutrient intake to support growth and health
- Feeding problems related to oral-motor and/or behavioral difficulties
- Medication-nutrient interactions
- Need for enteral (tube) feeding
- Chronic constipation or diarrhea
- Use of alternative or complementary therapies or products

This new pocket guide provides up-to-date and state-of-the art information on the tools and techniques for all aspects of nutrition care for CSHCN, while also incorporating the Nutrition Care Process. The reader may recognize that the content expands upon *Children with Special Health Care Needs: Nutrition Care Handbook* (2004) by including more information on the registered dietitian's role in early childhood intervention programs as well as in interdisciplinary team leadership during treatment of children with special health care needs. Updated references, additional case studies, and more distinctive tables for commonly used formulas in the nutrition care of children with special health care needs have also been provided in this new pocket guide.

Of course, not all topics can be condensed into a single pocket guide. For example, food-medication and herb-medication interactions are discussed in the pocket guide, but a comprehensive listing of interactions is not included because many other publications with extensive lists of all known food-medication and herb-medication interactions are available. Also, because manufacturers may alter and update formulary information, we have not attempted to include a comprehensive review of formula and supplemental products.

The *Academy of Nutrition and Dietetics Pocket Guide to Children with Special Health Care and Nutritional Needs* is a valuable tool for any health care professional working with this population, whether in clinical settings, management, or community dietetics. The goal of the editors and authors is to provide a quick-reference guide that covers the essential information needed for nutrition management of children with special health care needs. The guide will inspire a comprehensive, interdisciplinary approach to medical management of CSHCN. Up-to-date scientific evidence has been translated by the authors and editors into tables and easy-to-read guidelines for registered dietitians and other health care professionals to use in their daily practice.

Chapter 1

Growth

Jackie Krick, MS, RD,
Patricia Miller, MS, RD, CSP, and
Liz Enagonio, MS, RD, CNSC

INTRODUCTION TO GROWTH

Growth typically follows a predictable course. Growth potential is determined by genetics and is influenced by biological and environmental factors that can include disease, diet, and social and environmental circumstances. Early identification of growth problems is important because timely therapeutic interventions may positively affect a child's general health and functional abilities as well as supporting growth. Assessing growth is an integral component in examination of health. There can be both nutritional and non-nutritional reasons for different growth patterns. It is important to set realistic growth expectations for each individual child. Risk factors affecting growth in children with special health care needs are listed in Box 1.1.

Box 1.1   **Risk Factors Affecting Growth**

• Neuromotor performance • Cognition and communication skills • Problems with sensory input • Behavior/interaction • Growth retardation • Dietary adequacy • Gastrointestinal-related concerns • Abnormal tone and activity patterns • Positioning requirements • Increased incidence of scoliosis	• Increased incidence of seizures • Constipation • Amount of physical/verbal assistance needed • Physiological support • Oral motor skills/ swallowing • Medications • Dental and gum status • Multiple orthopedic procedures (increased incidence of scoliosis) • Family/psychosocial stressors • Dietary restrictions

IDEAL BODY WEIGHT

Ideal body weight (IBW) is the cornerstone to assess and monitor growth. Weight-for-stature and body mass index (BMI) are the measurement tools used to set IBW, as they do not rely on chronological age and they address proportionality. There are some children who follow their own curve for weight-for-age and height/length-for-age below the 5th percentile, which is acceptable as long as the BMI or weight-for-stature is within normal limits. The child who consistently plots below the 5th percentile but is growing along their established growth channel is of less concern than the child whose trajectory is trending down.

For children older than 3 years, minimally attaining and maintaining the 15th percentile weight-for-stature or BMI is sufficient to maintain health. This addresses caregiver concerns with respect to activities of daily living. Malnutrition is a primary concern during times of rapid cell growth and cell multiplication. This occurs from the prenatal period through age 2 years. An adequate diet is necessary during the period of rapid growth to achieve appropriate cell proliferation and reach optimal brain function. Achievement of normal rates of cell division can only occur if an adequate diet is re-established during the periods of rapid growth. Brain growth is most vulnerable from birth until 3 to 4 years of age at which point 90% of brain development has occurred. For children less than 3 years of age, setting the IBW minimally at the 25th to 50th percentile for weight-for-stature allows for brain growth and development irrespective of physical limitations. By 6 years of age, the brain is close to adult size and nutritional status may require re-evaluation (1,2).

Due to the chronicity of the underlying disorder, achieving IBW goals can be long term. In some instances, there might be a need for more rapid gains, such as pending surgical procedures, wound healing, and age. Factors to consider when determining IBW include:

- Age
- Actual vs expected rate of growth (use appropriate population- and/or diagnosis-specific data, if available)
- Analysis of longitudinal points
- Adequacy of fat and muscle stores
- Daily physical care and management (ADLs)
- Level of physical dependence
- Head circumference percentile
- Safety and efficiency of feeding
- General health status

GROWTH CHARTS

CDC Growth Charts/WHO Growth Standards

The Centers for Disease Control and Prevention (CDC) growth charts and World Health Organization (WHO) growth standards should be used only with careful interpretation, as children with special health care needs were not included in the reference population. The Maternal and Child Health Bureau provides an online training module that addresses the use of the CDC growth charts for children with special health care needs (http://depts .washington.edu/growth/cshcn/text/intro.htm).

The CDC recommends that the WHO growth standards be used to monitor growth for infants and children ages 0 to 2 years of age in the United States. The CDC growth charts are used for children and adolescents between 2 and 20 years of age. These growth charts allow for assessment of five growth indices: weight-for-age, stature- or length-for-age, weight-for-length, BMI-for-age, and head circumference for age. These charts are gender and age specific and can be used for children with a birth weight more than 1,500 g. The CDC growth charts and WHO Growth Standards can be downloaded from the CDC Web site (http://www.cdc.gov/growthcharts).

During preterm age, Fenton, and more recently Olsen, growth chart use is most appropriate. In 2003, Fenton conducted a meta-analysis of data from preterm infant population studies with a large sample size. Updated growth charts were created (3). In 2010, Olsen et al published data collected from 33 US states and 248 hospitals on infants ages 22 to 42 weeks (4). Table 1.1 provides guidelines for interpretation of growth in children with special health care needs using the CDC charts (5).

Table 1.1   Nutritional Status Indicators Using CDC Growth Charts

Anthropometric Index	Percentile Cut-Off Value (Nutritional Status Indicator)	Interpretation for Child With Special Health Care Needs[a]
BMI-for-age or Weight-for-length/ stature	>95th (Obesity)	• Common in Down syndrome or conditions that cause skeletal deformities such as spina bifida, scoliosis
BMI-for-age	>85th and <95th (Overweight)	• Common in conditions that limit ambulatory abilities
BMI-for-age or Weight-for-length	<5th (Underweight)	• Common in conditions that limit muscle mass such as spastic quadriplegia cerebral palsy • Common in feeding disorders • Common in conditions that affect absorption and metabolism
Stature/ length-for-age	>95th (Tall for age)	• Unusual, but characteristic of rare genetic disorders
Stature/ length-for-age	<5th (Short stature)	• Usually seen in neurologic disorders; microcephaly • May be related to prenatal factor or genetic disorder
Head circumference-for-age	>95th (Macrocephaly) <5th (Microcephaly)	• Developmental problems

Abbreviations: BMI, body mass index; CDC, Centers for Disease Control and Prevention.
[a]Interpretation related to children with special health care needs is based on clinical practice.
Source: Data are from reference 5.

Specialized Growth Charts

Many children with special health care needs have diagnoses for which there are no standardized growth charts; however, specialized charts are available for assessing growth of infants and children with certain conditions and syndromes. A full list with sources for obtaining the charts follows this section. These charts should be viewed as additional indices along with the CDC growth charts, as no single indicator should be used to assess a child's nutritional status. Clinical judgment should be integrated with objective data.

Concerns regarding the specialized charts relate to the small sample size used in their development, and they may not reflect the heterogeneity of specific populations. For example, in 2011 the American Academy of Pediatrics recommended against the use of existing specialty growth charts for Down syndrome; instead, standard CDC or WHO weight-for-height and BMI charts should be used with this population until revised research quality standards become available (6). In most cases, these specialty charts do not include all growth parameters and therefore lack the information to interpret weight/height or BMI or predict IBW. Box 1.2 features a list of specialty growth charts and where they can be located.

Box 1.2   Specialty Growth Charts

Preterm Growth Charts
- Casey PH, Kraemer HC, Bernbaum J, Tyson JE, Sells JC, Yogman MW, Bauer CR. Growth patterns of low birth weight preterm infants: a longitudinal analysis of a large, varied sample. *J Pediatr.* 1990;117:298–307.

(continued)

Box 1.2 Specialty Growth Charts (continued)

- Babson SG, Benda GI. Growth graphs for the clinical assessment of infants of varying gestational age. *J Pediatr.* 1976;89:815.
- Gairdner D, Peterson J. A growth chart for premature and other infants. *Arch Dis Child.* 1971;46:783–787.
- Fenton TR. A new growth chart for preterm babies: Babson and Benda's chart updated with recent data and a new format. *BMC Pediatr.* 2003;3:13.
- Olsen IE, Groveman SA, Lawson ML, et al. New intrauterine growth curves based on United States data. *Pediatrics.* 2010;125:e214–e224.

Achondroplasia
- Hoover-Fong JE, McGready J, Schultze KJ, Barnes H, Scott CI. Weight for age charts for children with achondroplasia. *Am J Med Genet.* 2007; 143A:2227–2235.
- Horton WA, Rotter JI, Rimoin DL, Scott CI, Hall JG. Standard growth curves for achondroplasia. *J Pediatr.* 1978;93:435–438.

Skeletal Dysplasias
- Genetics Education Center, University of Kansas Medical Center Web site. Dwarfism. http://www.kumc.edu/gec/support/dwarfism.html#growth.

Cerebral Palsy
- Krick J, Murphy-Miller P, Zeger S, Wright E. Pattern of growth in children with cerebral palsy. *J Am Diet Assoc.* 1996;96:680–685.
- Day SM. Growth patterns in a population of children and adolescents with cerebral palsy. *Dev Med Child Neurol.* 2007;49:167–171.
- Life Expectancy Project. Steven Day charts. http://www.lifeexpectancy.org/articles/GrowthCharts.shtml.

Cornelia de Lange Syndrome
- Klein DA, Barr M, Jackson, L. Growth manifestations in the Brachmann-deLange syndrome. *Am J Med Genet.* 1993;47:1042–1049.

(continued)

Box 1.2   Specialty Growth Charts (continued)

- Cornelia de Lange Syndrome Foundation. CdLS Growth Charts. http://www.cdlsusa.org/professional-education/treatment-protocols.htm. (Scroll down page to Growth section for links to charts for boys and girls.)

Down Syndrome
- Use standard weight-for-height or body mass index growth charts from the Centers for Disease Control and Prevention or World Health Organization until new research quality standards are developed (6).

Fragile X Syndrome
- Butler MG, Brunschwig A, Miller LK, Hagerman RJ. Standards for selected anthropometric measurements in males with the fragile X syndrome. *J Pediatr*. 1992;89:1059–1062.

Marfan Syndrome
- Erkula G, Jones KB, Sponseller PD, Dietz HC, Pyeritz RE. Growth and maturation in Marfan syndrome. *Am J Med Genet*. 2002;109:100–115.

Myelomeningocele
- Appendix 2. In: Ekvall S, ed. *Pediatric Nutrition in Chronic Disease and Developmental Disorders: Prevention, Assessment and Treatment*. New York, NY: Oxford Press; 1993.

Noonan Syndrome
- Witt DR, Keena BA, Hall JG, Allanson JE. Growth curves for height in Noonan syndrome. *Clin Genet*. 1986;30:150–153.
- The Noonan Syndrome Support Group. Noonan Syndrome Growth Charts. http://www.noonansyndrome.org/articles info/links.htm.

Prader-Willi Syndrome
- Butler MG, Sturich J, Lee J, Myers SE, Whitman BY, Gold JA, Kimonis V, Scheimann A, Terrazas N, Driscoll DJ. Growth standards of infants with Prader-Willi syndrome. *Pediatrics*. 2011;127:687–695.

(continued)

Box 1.2 Specialty Growth Charts (continued)

- Holm VA. Growth charts for Prader-Willi Syndrome. In: Greenswag LR and Alexander RC, eds. *Management of Prader-Willi Syndrome*. 2nd ed. New York, NY: Springer-Verlag; 1995.

Rubinstein-Taybi
- Stevens CA, Hennekam RC, Blackburn BL. Growth in the Rubinstein-Taybi syndrome. *Am J Med Genet*. 1990;6(suppl):51–55.

Sickle Cell Disease
- Phebus CK, Gloninger MF, Maciak BJ. Growth patterns by age and sex in children with sickle cell disease. *J Pediatr*. 1984;105:28–33.

Trisomy 13 and Trisomy 18
- Baty BJ, Blackburn BL, Carey JC. Natural history of tri-somy 18 and trisomy 13: I. Growth, physical assessment, medical histories, survival, and recurrence risk. *Am J Med Genet*. 1994;49:175–188.

Turner Syndrome
- Lyon AJ, Preece MA, Grant DB. Growth curve for girls with Turner syndrome. *Arch Dis Child*. 1985;60:932–935.

Williams Syndrome
- Morris CA, Demsey SA, Leonard CO, Dilts C, Blackburn BL. Natural history of Williams syndrome: physical charac-teristics. *J Pediatr*. 1988;113:318–326.
- Williams Syndrome Association. Growth Charts. http://www.williams-syndrome.org/search/node/growth+chart.

Growth Chart Collections
- Greenwood Genetic Center. *Growth References: Third Tri-mester to Adulthood*. 2nd ed. Greenwood, SC: Greenwood Genetic Center Publications; 1998. http://www.ggc.org/education/resources/ggc-publications/publications.html.
- University of Washington. Frequently Used Guidelines: Assessing Nutritional Status. Specialty Growth Charts. http://depts.washington.edu/nutrpeds/fug/growth/specialty.htm. Includes charts for a number of genetic conditions.

(continued)

Box 1.2   Specialty Growth Charts (continued)

> • The Magic Foundation. Growth Charts. http://www.magic
>   foundation.org/www/docs/7/growth-charts. Includes
>   growth charts for specific ethnic populations including
>   African-American, Caucasian, Chinese, Hispanic/Mexican-
>   American, Southeast Asian and Vietnamese children, as well
>   as children with genetic syndromes.
>
> **Interpretation of Growth Charts**
> • Centers for Disease Control and Prevention. CDC Growth
>   Charts. http://www.cdc.gov/growthcharts.
> • World Health Organization. The WHO Child Growth Stan-
>   dards. http://www.who.int/childgrowth/standards/en.

Enhancing Measurement Accuracy

It may be difficult to obtain accurate measurements in
children with contractures, scoliosis, or impaired tone.
Alternate methods for assessing stature include knee
height, upper arm length, or lower leg length. Reference
standards are available for children older than 2 years with
cerebral palsy (7). Arm span or total arm length can be
used to estimate stature for children who cannot stand.
Crown-rump length or sitting height measurements are
often useful estimates of stature for children with contractures of the lower body. These measurements will not
correlate directly with height or length, but can indicate
a child's rate of growth when plotted on CDC growth
charts. Although the measurements will be below the 5th
percentile for age, they will show whether or not the child
is following a consistent growth curve. These segmental
measurement techniques are described in references 2 and
8. It is important to use the same techniques for estimating
anthropometrics, especially stature, at each visit.

In the population of children with special health care needs, measurement errors are frequent. Potential errors can occur with the use of different scales in different settings; when subtracting the weight of a person holding the child; when converting between pounds and kilograms; and with incorrect technique, malfunctioning equipment, or lack of calibration.

Measurements should be consistent using the same scale, noting leg length discrepancy, without heavy clothing, bracing and/or splints, and well documented. When significant unexpected changes are seen repeating measurements is an important practice. Above all, clinical judgment should be used.

INCREMENTAL WEIGHT GAIN AND LINEAR GROWTH

Longitudinal data documents quantifiable rates of change that can be compared to reference data. Incremental weight gain and linear growth can be used to assess progress toward expected growth in children with special health care needs. When interventions are recommended, monitoring incremental changes evaluates not only the growth, but also the response to the nutritional therapy. Mean rates of growth for weight and stature are shown in Tables 1.2 through 1.5 (5). These rates of growth are representative of those children who follow along the 50th percentile. Therefore, it is acceptable for a child to grow at slower rates if they are consistently tracking along a satisfactory growth curve as determined by the clinician.

Table 1.2   Mean Daily Rates of Growth for Boys Birth to 24 Months[a]

Age, mo	Weight, g/d	Stature, cm/d
0–3	28	0.12
3–6	21	0.068
6–9	15	0.052
9–12	11	0.043
12–18	8	0.036
18–24	5	0.029

[a]Based on growth at the 50th percentile of the Centers for Disease Control and Prevention growth charts.
Source: Data are from reference 5.

Table 1.3   Mean Daily Rates of Growth for Girls Birth to 24 Months[a]

Age, mo	Weight, g/d	Stature, cm/d
0–3	24	0.11
3–6	19	0.067
6–9	14	0.051
9–12	11	0.043
12–18	8	0.037
18–24	5	0.030

[a]Based on growth at the 50th percentile of the Centers for Disease Control and Prevention growth charts.
Source: Data are from reference 5.

Table 1.4   Mean Monthly Rates of Weight Gain for Boys and Girls 3 to 20 Years[a]

Age, y	Boys, g/mo	Girls, g/mo
3–4	150	150
4–5	175	183
5–6	192	192
6–7	200	208
7–8	217	242
8–9	242	275
9–10	283	325
10–11	325	367
11–12	383	383
12–13	425	350
13–14	458	292
14–15	433	225
15–16	392	150
16–17	300	108
17–18	217	83
18–19	167	100
19–20	125	75

[a]Based on growth at the 50th percentile of the Centers for Disease Control and Prevention growth charts.
Source: Data are from reference 5.

Table 1.5   Mean Monthly Rates of Stature Gain for Boys and Girls 3 to 16 Years[a]

Age, y	Boys, cm/mo	Girls, cm/mo
3–4	0.6	0.5
4–5	0.5	0.6
5–6	0.6	0.6
6–7	0.5	0.6
7–8	0.5	0.5
8–9	0.5	0.4
9–10	0.4	0.4
10–11	0.4	0.5
11–12	0.5	0.7
12–13	0.6	0.5
13–14	0.6	0.25
14–15	0.5	0.08
15–16	0.3	0.08
16–17	0.2	0.08

[a]Based on growth at the 50th percentile of the Centers for Disease Control and Prevention growth charts.
Source: Data are from reference 5.

Z SCORES

Z scores for length-for-age, weight-for-age, weight-for-stature, and BMI provide an accurate evaluation of discreet changes from one measure to another. Percentile tables typically describe ranges, and consequently detection of movement within the range is difficult to describe. The z score denotes standard deviation units from the median and is more precise than percentile ranges. See Box 1.3 for questions to consider in establishing a schedule to monitor growth. Programs available online to calculate z scores can be found on the CDC Epi Info Web site (www.cdc.gov/epiinfo) and from StatCoder (www.statcoder.com).

Box 1.3   Questions to Consider when Establishing a Schedule to Monitor Growth

- Is the child following a saw tooth pattern or showing consistent desired growth?
- Is the child less than 3 years of age or older?
- Is the child failing to thrive or gaining too rapidly?
- Are financial resources strained?
- Are there significant emotional stressors for the patient and/or patient's family?
- Are there conflicting opinions/recommendations from other health care providers causing confusion?
- Is compliance with nutrition recommendations a concern?
- Are there pending hospitalizations/surgeries?
- Is access to care a concern?

BODY COMPOSITION

Muscle, adipose tissue, and bone change during growth. There are a number of methods for assessing fat mass, fat free or lean mass, and bone density. They may be used as adjuncts to stature and weight measurements.

Skinfold Thickness and Arm Circumference

Skinfold thickness and arm circumference can provide a more comprehensive picture of the child's nutritional status (9). It should be noted that the accuracy of arm circumference and skinfold measurements depends on frequent calibration of the instruments and the experience of the person taking measurements. Various physiological conditions including hydration status and muscle tone affect the compressibility of tissues; therefore, information derived from anthropometry should be used in conjunction with clinical observations and biochemical studies. Skinfold and arm circumference can be monitored using the child as his/her own control to determine trends (10).

Bone Growth

Skeletal maturation occurs within a predictable sequence of events including fusion of the epiphyses and the appearance of ossification centers. Acquisition of bone mass continues until around age 25 years. Bone age is often used to evaluate a child whose linear growth is proceeding at an unusual rate. In children, bone mass is assessed against age-related z scores. Delayed or accelerated bone growth can be used for diagnosis of certain syndromes or to estimate the potential for catch-up growth. Bone or skeletal age is usually measured by an x-ray of the hand and wrist.

Building a lifetime calcium reserve is an important aspect of skeletal growth. Children with low bone mass are at increased risk for fractures and osteoporosis. A dual energy x-ray absorptiometry (DEXA) scan can assess bone mineralization, and may be helpful in identifying and treating children with low bone mass. Because there are a number of factors that influence bone mass and because there are numerous normative data sets, interpretation requires clinical correlation (11). In children, a diagnosis of low bone mass should not be made on the basis of DEXA alone, but must be considered in relation to biochemical tests, other anthropometrics, gender, ethnicity, and medical diagnoses. The biochemical tests include serum albumin/pre-albumin, calcium, phosphorus, alkaline phosphatase, and 25(OH) vitamin D. Urine calcium excretion mirrors calcium absorption and vitamin D status and can be assessed using a random morning, second void specimen. The following parameters affect bone growth:

- Gender
- Body size
- Dietary adequacy
- Family history
- Age
- Weight bearing status
- Ethnicity
- Level of physical mobility
- Medications (eg, anticonvulsants, corticosteroids)

Specialized Methods for Assessing Body Composition

Bioelectric impedance (BIA) estimates body fat, lean body mass, and total body water through the difference in electrical conductivity in fat vs fat free tissues. Its interpretation is affected by hydration status and several medical conditions (2). BIA is not commonly used in a clinical setting. Doubly labeled water (D_2O) uses the dilution of a labeled isotope of hydrogen to measure total body water and estimate fat-free mass. Its use is confined primarily to research facilities.

ETHICAL CONSIDERATIONS

Parents often voice concerns regarding home management for their children as they grow in size and weight, and at times may limit dietary intake to stop the progress of growth. An extreme example of this involves growth attenuation (12). It involves children with profound disabilities who typically have permanent, limited cognitive skills and require total care by others. Clinicians practicing in the field of developmental disabilities should be aware of this issue. Ethics committees in pediatric hospitals can help to mediate difficult controversial conversations within an ethical context where all values are respected and heard.

APPLICABLE ICD-9 CODES

The International Statistical Classification of Diseases and Related Health Problems (ICD) codes are used for billing purposes. These codes are in the public domain and easily accessed online (13). Below is a list of industry-wide accepted billing ICD-9 codes related to growth to assist clinicians in private practice and outpatient clinics:

- 783: Symptoms concerning nutrition, metabolism, and development
- 783.1: Abnormal weight gain (excludes obesity)
- 783.2: Abnormal loss of weight and underweight
- 783.21: Loss of weight
- 783.22: Underweight
- 783.41: Failure to thrive/Failure to gain weight
- 783.43: Short stature, which is defined by constitutional short stature; stature inconsistent with chronological age.

Note: Effective January 2013, ICD-10 codes will replace ICD-9 codes. See reference 13 for additional information.

SUMMARY

When addressing or assessing growth, remember the following points:

- Growth is the outcome measure that corroborates the efficacy of nutrition interventions. Growth plays a role in decisions regarding nutrition support, the timing of surgical or medical interventions, and in modifying or replacing assistive equipment.
- Actual or ideal body weight is the basis for decisions related to energy needs, fluid needs, and medication doses.
- Monitoring growth will provide feedback to interdisciplinary team members who are implementing therapeutic interventions.
- Growth goals provide a reference point for parents/ caregivers, and may be used as a teaching and monitoring tool.
- Assessing adequate growth requires objective clinical tools, as well as clinical judgment.
- While the desired weight changes over time, attaining and maintaining an adequate growth goal percentile provides a long-term achievement.

When thinking specifically about growth, it is helpful to address the needs of three separate, but connected groups: the child, the family, and the community. Achieving reasonable growth goals enables the child to participate to his or her full capacity in the learning and therapeutic environments. Family understanding and support will provide the best assistance for the patient. Additionally, community collaboration and coordination will help a child achieve these clearly defined goals.

REFERENCES

1. Hervada A, Hervada-Page M. Brain development and the critical period of brain growth. In: Lifshitz F, ed. *Childhood Nutrition*. Boca Raton, FL. CRC Press; 1995.

2. Ekvall SW, Ekvall VK, Walberg-Wolfe J, Nehring W. Nutritional assessment—all levels and ages. In: Ekvall SW, Ekvall VK, eds. *Pediatric Nutrition in Chronic Diseases and Developmental Disorders; Prevention, Assessment, and Treatment*. 2nd ed. New York, NY: Oxford University Press; 2005:47–48; 50–51;477–481.

3. Fenton TR. A new growth chart for preterm babies: Babson and Benda's chart updated with recent data and a new format. *BMC Pediatr*. 2003;3:13.

4. Olsen IE, Groveman SA, Lawson ML, et al. New intrauterine growth curves based on United States data. *Pediatrics*. 2010; 125:e214–e224.

5. Centers for Disease Control and Prevention. Use and Interpretation of CDC Growth Charts. http://www.cdc.gov/nccdphp/dnpa/growthcharts/guide_intro.htm. Accessed August 24, 2009.

6. Wyckoff AS. AAP updates guidance on caring for children with Down syndrome. *AAP News*. 2011;32(8). www.aapnews.org. Accessed October 10, 2011.

7. Spender QW, Cronk CE, Charney EB, Stallings VA. Assessment of linear growth of children with cerebral palsy: use of alternative measures to height or length. *Dev Med Child Neurol*. 1989; 31:206–214.

8. American Academy of Pediatrics. Nutritional support for children with developmental disabilities. In: *Pediatric Nutrition Handbook*. 6th ed. Elk Grove Village, IL; American Academy of Pediatrics; 2009:821–842.

9. Zemel B, Stallings V. Energy requirements and nutritional assessment in developmental disabilities. In: Walker WA, Watkins JB, eds. *Nutrition in Pediatrics*. Hamilton, ON: BD Decker; 1996:169–177.

10. Samour P, King K. *Handbook of Pediatric Nutrition*. 3rd ed. Sudbury, MA: Jones and Bartlett; 2005:12.

11. Binkovitz LA, Henwood MJ. Pediatric DXA: technique and interpretation. *Pediatr Radiol*. 2007;37:21–23.

12. Gunther F, Diekema D. Attenuating growth in children with profound developmental disability. *Arch Pediatr Adolesc Med.* 2006;160:1013–1017.

13. Centers for Disease Control and Prevention. Classification of Diseases, Functioning and Disability. http://www.cdc .gov/nchs/icd.htm. Accessed June 15, 2011.

Chapter 2

Diet and Nutrition

Sharon C. Weston, MS, RD, and
Patricia Murray, MEd, RD

OVERVIEW OF NUTRITION SCREENING AND FOOD/ NUTRITION-RELATED NUTRITION ASSESSMENT

The process of screening for nutrition and feeding issues is essential for any health care team and should be the first step involved in a nutritional status evaluation (1). Many screening instruments are used for identification of nutrition concerns. Routine screening criteria include age, anthropometrics, clinical observations (such as skin, hair, fingernails, and dental concerns), medical history, laboratory values, diet history, and feeding ability. Ideally, screening is simple to administer, and can be performed by a variety of health care professionals (see Table 2.1) (2–5). Based on the information provided by the screening tool, nutritional risk is evaluated.

Table 2.1 Screening for Nutrition and Feeding Issues in Children

Area of Focus	Nutritional Risk Factors: Refer if . . .
Concerns about food intake, feeding difficulties, and feeding and oral motor concerns	Inadequate or inappropriate dietary intake for more than 3 days; delay in developmental feeding skills

(continued)

**Table 2.1   Screening for Nutrition and Feeding Issues
in Children** (continued)

Area of Focus	Nutritional Risk Factors: Refer if . . .
Child's typical feeding pattern (types of foods eaten and how often)	Alternative or special diet (vegan, multiple food allergies, etc); consumes only liquids, pureed foods, or ground foods after age 2 years; pica (intake of nonfood items)
Fluid and bowel problems	Inadequate fluid intake; constipation; diarrhea; dehydration
Use of nutritional supplements	Used on a regular basis for supplementation of the diet
Use of vitamin/mineral supplements	Use of supplements exceeding 100% DRIs/ULs without physician approval
Use of complementary/ alternative nutritional therapies	Intentional omission of a food group (such as dairy); unproven herbal supplementation
Adequacy of food resources and participation in eligible food and nutrition programs	Inadequate food supply; financial difficulties

Abbreviations: DRI, Dietary Reference Intake; UL, Tolerable Upper Intake Level.
Source: Data are from references 2–5.

A thorough nutrition assessment is necessary if a child is screened as nutritionally at risk. The nutrition assessment is the basis for making nutrition diagnoses and determining appropriate nutrition interventions. The process of assessing the intake of a child with special health care needs is the same as assessing any other child. There are, however, additional areas to review. Tables 2.2 and 2.3 identify information that should be obtained in a general pediatric nutrition assessment of food/nutrition-related history and includes special considerations that should be noted when completing a nutrition assessment for a child with special health care needs (2). Box 2.1 provides clinical tips regarding the use of food diaries.

Table 2.2   Nutrition Assessment of Food Intake

Information to Obtain for All Pediatric Clients	*Special Considerations for Children with Special Needs*
Type, brand name, and amount of food, beverages, or formula actually consumed at a meal or snack	Child may lose food from mouth due to oral–motor feeding problems or vomiting; may be helpful to observe a meal or snack.
Preparation methods for foods and formula	Recipes may be modified by addition of fat, sugars, or protein. Request exact recipe for formula, including ingredients, amounts, preparation methods, and storage.
Favorite foods, food dislikes, food jags, food allergies, food intolerances, lack of dietary variety with regards to solids	Determine how eating patterns and intake are altered when the child is ill or when there is a change in the medical condition or medication (eg, child refuses to eat or reduced fluid intake).
Frequency, length, and location of meals and snacks	Obtain food diaries (both weekdays and weekend); determine how many people feed the child throughout the day; observe an actual meal or snack.
Child's independence in obtaining food	If the child is dependent on others to be fed, determine whether the feeders can identify hunger and fullness.
Current and past use of nutrition supplements or special diets	May indicate nutritional risk or a history of nutritional risk from a medical condition.
Fluid intake and bowel habits	Constipation, diarrhea, dehydration due to low tone, medications, excessive drooling, feeding difficulties, or medical conditions.

Source: Data are from reference 3.

**Table 2.3   Nutrition Assessment of Factors that Influence
Food Intake**

Information to Obtain for All Pediatric Clients	Special Considerations for Children with Special Needs
Cultural or ethnic family eating practices	Determine family's beliefs and values regarding feeding a child with a disability or special health care needs.
Use of complementary/ alternative nutrition therapies including restrictive diets	Determine if and how this affects the child's food intake and nutritional adequacy; determine exact amounts of supplements, cost as well as safety.
Activity level or ambulation	Affects energy needs if child is overactive or limited in mobility.
Pertinent eating/feeding history	Determine whether feeding history correlates with the child's advancement in other areas of development.
Parent's perception of the role of nutrition/feeding practices as they relate to the child's health condition	Helps determine the degree of knowledge and/or stress parents/caregivers may be experiencing with their child's eating/ feeding or growth.
Caregiver's ability to recognize hunger and satiety cues	Lack of awareness may alter the child's intake (either feeding more or less than required).
Other programs or therapies that may be providing food as a reward/therapy	If close to mealtimes, may affect a child's intake.
Use of nonoral enteral feeding	Refer to Chapter 4.

Source: Data are from reference 3.

Box 2.1   Clinical Tip: Food Diaries

Food diaries are essential in any assessment of nutrient intake.
Although food diaries may be difficult for parents and caregivers to complete, they can provide the registered dietitian
(RD) with a wealth of information that forms the basis of their
evaluation of dietary intake and indicates strategies for optimal nutritional management. Food diaries should include the
following information:

- Time and length of meal
- Location
- Who fed or prepared the food (specifically if the child is
  dependent on these activities)
- Food and drinks offered and what was refused
- Food and drinks consumed
- Food and drinks lost from mouth
- Wherever possible the ingredients in the food
- Use and consumption of medications or supplements

Occasionally, it is also helpful to note how the child was feeling before and after meals. This may include physiological
changes such as energy status or stomach pains. It is also helpful to describe if the day recorded was "typical" or unusual in
some way, the child's general health, and physical activities
during the day. Because caregivers may over– or underreport,
the RD should review the food diary and verify the portions
with measuring cups, spoons, bottles, and food models when-
ever possible. The most common errors are omitting liquids
and small snacks between scheduled meal times. Having the
parent/caregiver relate eating with the day's activities is a
good way to help them remember small snacks and fluids consumed. If the child is also experiencing issues with diarrhea,
vomiting, or constipation, or altered behavior at meals, this
information should also be recorded in the food diary. It may
benefit the RD to have pictures of the plate taken so as that he
or she can better evaluate serving sizes.

NUTRITION ASSESSMENT OF
MEDICAL/HEALTH HISTORY

A child's medical history can have a direct (primary) or indirect (secondary) effect on the child's overall growth and development. Boxes 2.2 through 2.11 can be used as a guide when assessing children with a known diagnosis (1,3,4,6). Some children may not exhibit all or any of the identified risk factors at the time of the assessment, but the problem may arise later.

Box 2.2   Attention Deficit/Hyperactivity Disorder: Frequently Reported Nutrition Problems/Factors Contributing to Nutritional Risk

- Possibly underweight due to side effects of certain medications
- Disruptive mealtimes if untreated
- Certain medications can decrease appetite

Source: Data are from references 1, 3, 4, and 6.

Box 2.3   Autism: Frequently Reported Nutrition Problems/ Factors Contributing to Nutritional Risk

- GI issues
- Limited food selection
- Sensory feeding/eating problems
- Behavioral eating/feeding problems
- Pica
- Medication–nutrient interactions

Source: Data are from references 1, 3, 4, and 6.

Box 2.4 Cerebral Palsy: Frequently Reported Nutrition Problems/Factors Contributing to Nutritional Risk

- Growth problems
- Failure to thrive
- Overweight due to hypotonia
- Gastrointestinal issues
- Oral–motor problems
- Central nervous system involvement
- Orthopedic problems
- Medication–nutrient interactions related to seizure disorder

Source: Data are from references 1, 3, 4, and 6.

Box 2.5 Cleft Lip/Palate: Frequently Reported Nutrition Problems/Factors Contributing to Nutritional Risk

- Underweight/failure to thrive
- Requires use of special nipples if bottle feeding
- Feedings may be lengthy
- Lactation support may be warranted if breast feeding

Source: Data are from references 1, 3, 4, and 6.

Box 2.6 Congenital Heart Disease: Frequently Reported Nutrition Problems/Factors Contributing to Nutritional Risk

- Underweight/failure to thrive prior to corrective surgeries
- Increased energy needs
- Gastrointestinal issues
- Poor feeding and fatigue prior to surgery
- Medications may decrease appetite

Source: Data are from references 1, 3, 4, and 6.

Box 2.7 Cystic Fibrosis: Frequently Reported Nutrition Problems/Factors Contributing to Nutritional Risk

- Underweight
- Increased nutrient needs
- Decreased food intake
- Decreased absorption of nutrients related to pancreatic insufficiency and chronic pulmonary infection
- GI issues
- Increase in secondary illnesses: diabetes, liver disease, osteoporosis

Source: Data are from references 1, 3, 4, and 6.

Box 2.8 Down Syndrome: Frequently Reported Nutrition Problems/Factors Contributing to Nutritional Risk

- Risk for obesity
- Altered energy needs related to short stature and hypotonia
- Gastrointestinal issues
- Poor suck in infancy
- Gum disease
- Increased risk for heart disease, osteoporosis, and Alzheimer's disease

Source: Data are from references 1, 3, 4, and 6.

Box 2.9 Prader–Willi Syndrome: Frequently Reported Nutrition Problems/Factors Contributing to Nutritional Risk

- High risk for obesity
- Failure to thrive in infancy; later obesity related to hypotonia and short stature
- Gastrointestinal issues
- Poor suck in infancy
- Behavioral feeding/eating problems
- Risk for diabetes mellitus

Source: Data are from references 1, 3, 4, and 6.

**Box 2.10   Seizure Disorder: Frequently Reported Nutrition
Problems/Factors Contributing to Nutritional Risk**

- GI issues
- Certain medications that alter absorption or utilization of
  nutrients

Source: Data are from references 1, 3, 4, and 6.

**Box 2.11   Spina Bifida (Myelomeningocele): Frequently
Reported Nutrition Problems/Factors Contributing to
Nutritional Risk**

- Risk for obesity
- Decreased energy needs based on short stature and limited
  mobility
- Constipation
- Swallowing problems caused by the Arnold Chiari malfor-
  mation of the brain
- Urinary tract infections

Source: Data are from references 1, 3, 4, and 6.

NUTRITION ASSESSMENT OF DIETARY INTAKE

Nutrition assessment involves determining the nutrient
intake of the child and comparing this intake to standards.
Although commonly accepted guidelines for determining
the dietary intake for infants and children exist (6,7), it is
important to take into account the individual child's needs.
For example, the chronological and developmental age of
the child may affect dietary progression (see Box 2.12
for information on typical progression). Altered energy
needs may impact serving sizes. Specific medical conditions may restrict certain food groups and increase the use
of other foods or supplements as a replacement. Box 2.13
offers clinical tips related to food intake (8). See Chapter
3 for more detailed information about feeding concerns.

Box 2.12 Typical Feeding Progression and Serving Sizes for Healthy Infants and Toddlers

Ages 0–4 Months: Breastmilk and/or formula: 8–12 servings/d (typical serving size: 2–4 oz)

Ages 4–6 Months
- Breastmilk and/or formula: 4–6 servings/d (typical serving size: 6–8 oz)
- Grains (iron–fortified infant cereal): 1–2 servings/d (typical serving size: 1–2 Tbsp)

Ages 6–8 Months
- Breastmilk and/or formula: 3–5 servings/d (typical serving size: 6–8 oz)
- Grains (iron–fortified infant cereal; crackers): 2 servings/d (typical serving sizes: 2–4 Tbsp cereal; 2 crackers)
- Fruits and vegetables: 2 servings/d—1 serving 100% juice diluted with equal amount of water; 1 serving fruit or vegetable (typical serving sizes: 3 oz diluted juice; 2–3 Tbsp fruit or vegetable)

Ages 8–12 Months
- Breastmilk and/or formula, dairy foods (cheese; yogurt): 3–4 servings/d (typical serving sizes: 6–8 oz breastmilk/formula; ½ oz cheese; ½ cup yogurt)
- Grains (iron–fortified infant cereal; bread; crackers; pasta): 2 servings/d (typical serving sizes: 2–4 Tbsp cereal; ½ slice bread; 2 crackers; 3–4 Tbsp pasta)
- Fruits and vegetables: 3 servings/d—2 servings fruit or vegetable; 1 serving juice (typical serving sizes: 3–4 Tbsp fruit or vegetable; 2–3 oz juice in a cup)
- Protein (chicken; beef; pork; legumes): 2 servings/d (typical serving size: 3–4 Tbsp)

Ages 12–24 Months
- Dairy (whole milk; cheese; yogurt): 3 servings/d (typical serving sizes: 4 oz milk; ½ oz cheese; ½ cup yogurt)
- Grain (cereal; pasta; rice; bread; crackers): 4 servings/d (typical serving sizes: ¼ cup cereal, pasta, or rice; ½ slice bread; 2 crackers)

(continued)

**Box 2.12   Typical Feeding Progression and Serving Sizes for
               Healthy Infants and Toddlers** (continued)

Ages 12–24 Months (continued)
- Fruits and vegetables (all types): 4 servings/d (typical serving size: ¼ cup cooked or raw)
- Protein (chicken; beef; pork; legumes; eggs): 2 servings/d (typical serving size: 1 oz meat; ¼ cup legumes; 1 egg)

Source: Data are from reference 6.

Box 2.13   Clinical Tips: Food Intake

- A good rule for recommended serving sizes is 1 Tbsp of each of the food groups per age, per meal.
- High intake of juice early in life has been associated with dental caries and reduced intake of other nutrients (protein, fat, iron, etc). The American Academy of Pediatrics (AAP) recommends that juices be provided to infants 6 months of age or older or when they can drink from a cup. AAP also recommends no more than 4 to 6 oz of 100% juice per day as part of a meal or snack for children ages 1 to 6 years. Juice can be diluted to 50% juice 50% water. For older children and adolescents ages 7 to 18 years, the AAP recommends the maximum of 8 to 12 oz of juice per day (8).
- Infants and children who have a family history of allergies may be advised by their pediatrician to avoid foods commonly associated with severe allergic reactions. When introducing new foods, it is recommended to wait approximately 3 to 5 days before introducing another new food in order to monitor for signs of intolerance. *See* Food Hypersensitivities section of this chapter for more information.
- Clinical judgment is needed when recommending the introduction of solid foods to infants and children who have oral–motor or sensory feeding problems. Recommending ways to adapt how a food is prepared or presented is important.

                                                              (continued)

Box 2.13   Clinical Tips: Food Intake (continued)

- Baby foods should not be added to infant formula or put in a bottle. However, due to feeding difficulties, pureed baby foods may be used to thicken liquids as recommended by a feeding specialist.
- Between 12 and 24 months of age, a child's appetite decreases and this will often alarm parents. It is important to reassure parents this decrease is normal because the child's rate of growth has slowed considerably. Small, frequent, and nutrient–dense foods are needed at this age. The manner in which the food is presented to a child is also important. The use of different colors and shapes can encourage a child to eat a variety of nutritious foods. Appropriate portions should be used so that parents do not overwhelm, or alternatively, overfeed the child.

USE OF DIETARY REFERENCE INTAKES

The Institute of Medicine's Dietary Reference Intakes (DRIs) are a set of nutrient-based reference values that were developed in response to a need for a more precise and customized approach to defining nutrient requirements. The DRIs are composed of four different estimates regarding recommendations for the long-term health and well-being of a population. These estimations are in the form of the following:

- Estimated Average Requirement (EAR)
- Recommended Dietary Allowance (RDA)
- Adequate Intake (AI)
- Tolerable Upper Intake Level (UL)
- Estimated Energy Requirement (EER)

The goal of the DRIs is to describe nutrient requirements for the prevention or delay of chronic diseases.

Health care providers can obtain more information about
DRIs as well as the summary tables from the Food and
Nutrition Information Center of the National Agriculture
Library (http://fnic.nal.usda.gov). The full DRI publica-
tions are available from the National Academies Press
Web site (http://nap.edu).

MEASURING OR ESTIMATING ENERGY REQUIREMENTS

Understanding and assessing energy requirements is a
challenge in the clinical setting. One of the most accurate
methods to measure energy expenditure involves indirect calorimetry, a method of measuring gas exchanges.
Another accurate method utilizes doubly labeled water
to determine carbohydrate production. Although highly
accurate, this method is used mostly in research settings.
Both methods are time consuming and usually impractical
in the clinical setting.

Equations

Various equations have been developed to estimate energy
requirements in clinical and research settings. In addition
to EER, these calculations include, but are not limited to,
the Harris-Benedict, Schofield, and World Health Organization (WHO) equations (6). The WHO equation does
not require a linear measurement, which makes it useful
in estimating energy needs for patients whose heights
are difficult to obtain. Clinical judgment is used to determine the appropriate equation to use and child's degree
of activity.

Calculating the EER for boys and girls ages 3 to 19
years involves using age-appropriate equations and insert-
ing the most appropriate physical activity coefficient

(PA) into the equation. The PA varies by age, sex, and the degree of activity (9). Equations for determining EER in infants and healthy weight children and adolescents as well as Total Energy Expenditure (TEE) for overweight boys and girls ages 3 to 19 years are available (9). TEE can be used by clinicians as an estimate of energy expenditure with the goal of weight loss, weight maintenance or weight gain. See Tables 2.4, 2.5, and 2.6 for EER and TEE equations (9). As physical activity is variable, their PA is also variable. Tables 2.7 and 2.8 provide suggestions for estimated PA coefficients (9). See Table 2.9 for Resting Energy Expenditure (REE) equations and Table 2.10 for stress factors (6). Note that children with special health care needs have differing energy requirements. Equations must be used in conjunction with clinical judgment. Growth should be monitored and adjustments in energy intake should be made based on weight goals (10).

Table 2.4   Estimated Energy Requirements for Infants and Young Children

Age, mo	EER, kcal/d
0–3	$(89 \times Wt - 100) + 175$
4–6	$(89 \times Wt - 100) + 56$
7–12	$(89 \times Wt - 100) + 22$
13–35	$(89 \times Wt - 100) + 20$

Abbreviations: EER, Estimated Energy Requirement; Wt, weight (kg).
Source: Data are from reference 9.

Table 2.5 Estimated Energy Requirements and Total Energy Expenditure for Boys

Age, y	Equation
3–8	EER = $88.5 - 61.9 \times \text{Age [y]} + \text{PA} \times (26.7 \times \text{Wt} + 903 \times \text{Ht}) + 20$
9–18	EER = $88.5 - 61.9 \times \text{Age [y]} + \text{PA} \times (26.7 \times \text{Wt} + 903 \times \text{Ht}) + 25$
3–18, overweight	TEE = $114 - 50.9 \times \text{Age [y]} + \text{PA} \times (19.5 \times \text{Wt} + 1161.4 \times \text{Ht})$

Abbreviations: EER, Estimated Energy Requirement (kcal/d); Ht, height (meters); PA, physical activity coefficient; TEE, Total Energy Expenditure (kcal/d); Wt, weight (kg).
Source: Data are from reference 9.

Table 2.6 Estimated Energy Requirements and Total Energy Expenditure for Girls

Age, y	Equation
3–8	EER = $135.3 - 30.8 \times \text{Age [y]} + \text{PA} \times (10.0 \times \text{Wt} + 934 \times \text{Ht}) + 20$
9–18	EER = $135.3 - 30.8 \times \text{Age [y]} + \text{PA} \times (10.0 \times \text{Wt} + 934 \times \text{Ht}) + 25$
3–18, overweight	TEE = $389 - 41.2 \times \text{Age [y]} + \text{PA} \times (15.0 \times \text{Wt} + 701 \times \text{Ht})$

Abbreviations: EER, Estimated Energy Requirement (kcal/d); Ht, height (meters); PA, physical activity coefficient; TEE, Total Energy Expenditure (kcal/d); Wt, weight (kg).
Source: Data are from reference 9.

Table 2.7   Physical Activity (PA) Coefficients for Boys Ages 3 to 18 Years

Activity Level	Coefficient	
	Normal Weight	Overweight
Sedentary	1.00	1.00
Low active	1.13	1.12
Active	1.26	1.24
Very active	1.42	1.45

Source: Data are from reference 9.

Table 2.8   Physical Activity (PA) Coefficients for Girls Ages 3 to 18 Years

Activity Level	Coefficient	
	Normal Weight	Overweight
Sedentary	1.00	1.00
Low active	1.16	1.18
Active	1.31	1.35
Very active	1.56	1.60

Source: Data are from reference 9.

Table 2.9   World Health Organization Equations for Estimating Resting Energy Expenditures

Age, y	REE for Males	REE for Females
0–3	$(60.9 \times Wt) - 54$	$(60.1 \times Wt) - 51$
3–10	$(22.7 \times Wt) + 495$	$(22.5 \times Wt) + 499$
10–18	$(17.5 \times Wt) + 651$	$(12.2 \times Wt) + 746$

Abbreviations: REE, Resting Energy Expenditure (kcal/d); Wt, Weight (kg).
Source: Data are from reference 6.

Table 2.10 Stress Factors and Effects on Energy Requirements

Type of Stress	Multiply REE by
Starvation	0.70–0.85
Surgery	1.05–1.5
Sepsis	1.2–1.6
Closed head injury	1.3
Trauma	1.1–1.8
Growth failure	1.5–2.0
Burn	1.5–2.5

Source: Data are from reference 6.

Calculating Energy Requirements in Children with Special Health Care Needs

As stated previously, children with special needs often do not conform to the standard equations. Additional equations are available to be used to assess patient's needs. It is essential to use these in conjunction with anthropometric, biochemical, and clinical assessments along with a thorough exam of diet history and clinical judgment. Standard methods for determining energy requirements for children with special health care needs are used to begin an assessment, but alterations may be necessary due to the child's medical diagnosis. Box 2.14 can be used as a guide to determine estimated energy requirements (9).

**Box 2.14 Alternative Methods of Estimating Daily Energy
Requirements Based on Health Condition**

Down Syndrome
- 14.3 kcal/cm for girls ages 5–11 years
- 16.1 kcal/cm for boys ages 5–11 years

Spina Bifida
Children older than 8 years who are minimally active:
- To maintain weight: 9–11 kcal/cm, or 50% fewer kcal
  than recommended for a child of the same age without the
  condition
- To promote weight loss: 7 kcal/cm

Prader–Willi Syndrome
For all children and adolescents:
- 10–11 kcal/cm to maintain growth within a growth channel
- 8.5 kcal/cm for slow weight loss and support linear growth

Cerebral Palsy
- Ambulatory, ages 5–12 years: 13.9 kcal/cm
- Nonambulatory, ages 5–12 years: 11.1 kcal/cm
- Cerebral palsy with severely restricted activity: 10 kcal/cm
- Cerebral palsy with mild to moderate activity: 15 kcal/cm

Failure to Thrive
Energy requirement will depend on etiology or medical condition, but start with EER calculations using ideal body weight
for height–age and EER for height–age. *Height–age* is defined
as age at which current height or length would fall at the 50th
percentile on the height–for–age or length–for–age growth
chart (*see* Chapter 1). *Ideal body weight for height–age* is
defined as weight at the 50th percentile for height–age.
Example: A 9–month–old old girl with weight of 6.4 kg and
length of 66 cm (height–age = 6 months). Ideal body weight
for a 6–month–old girl is 7.3 kg.

$$\text{EER (kcal/d)} = (89 \times \text{Weight [kg]} - 100) + 56$$
$$= (89 \times 7.3 - 100) + 56$$
$$= 606$$

(continued)

**Box 2.14   Alternative Methods of Estimating Daily Energy
            Requirements Based on Health Condition** (continued)

To calculate estimated catch–up growth needs, use the following formula:

Energy needs (kcal/d) = (EER for Age × Ideal Weight for
                        Height [kg])/Actual Weight (kg)

Cystic Fibrosis
Calculate ideal weight based on height, using the pediatric
growth chart. Multiply by the child's EER for age. Multiply by
a factor of 1.3–1.5 (depending on the severity of the disease) to
compensate for increased energy demands.

Abbreviation: EER, Estimated Energy Requirement (*see* Tables 2.4–2.6).
Source: Data are from references 6 and 9.

NUTRITION ASSESSMENT OF MACRONUTRIENT
AND MICRONUTRIENT INTAKE

Macronutrients

The macronutrient distribution (carbohydrate, protein,
and fat as a percentage of total energy intake) of an infant
or child's diet must be calculated and compared to the distribution
requirements as set by the DRIs (see Table 2.11)
(9). An unbalanced diet can result in short- or long-term
complications. For example, a high percentage of fat in a
formula can result in delayed gastric emptying, reflux, and
discomfort for the child. Alternatively, inadequate fat can
lead to essential fatty acid deficiency. Specialized diets put
patients at an increased risk of imbalances of macronutrient
distribution. Special care must be taken to assess and
monitor the macronutrients as they pertain to individual
diseases and the complications that relate to it.

Table 2.11   Acceptable Macronutrient Distribution Ranges

Age	Range, % of energy		
	Carbohydrate	*Fat*	*Protein*
Full–term infant	35–65	30–55	7–16
1–3 y	45–65	30–40	5–20
4–18 y	45–65	25–35	10–30

Source: Data are from reference 9.

Micronutrients

Micronutrient intake should be compared to the DRIs for age. Special consideration should be taken to ensure adequate vitamin and mineral intake levels be met for children on restrictive or hypocaloric diets. Drug-nutrient interactions, which will be discussed later in this chapter, may also interfere with vitamin/mineral levels and should be taken into account.

ESTIMATION OF FLUID REQUIREMENTS AND FIBER NEEDS

Maintaining adequate hydration is important for over-all fluid balance within the body as well as prevention of bowel problems. Maintaining appropriate hydration in children with special health care needs is particularly challenging. These children occasionally experience fluid losses from drooling, poor oral control when drinking, or losses from tubes or wounds. Additionally, those children who are dependent on others for feeding or who have difficulty communicating dehydration require additional attention. They may be embarrassed to ask to relieve themselves frequently or attempt to avoid the discomfort related to soiled diapers. Additionally, patients with cystic fibrosis have increased fluid (and electrolyte) needs because of the increased losses during sweating. Some children might have difficulty swallowing thinner liquids so it is more difficult to achieve goal volumes. Children with special health care needs may encounter bowel problems more frequently due to low tone, withholding, and specialized diets. In certain cases, a child may need an evaluation from a speech or occupational therapist familiar with swallowing risks to assess the safety of drinking liquids without the risk of aspiration.

Fluid Needs

The estimation of fluid needs can be calculated using the Holliday-Segar Method, as outlined in Table 2.12 (6). Promoting a fluid-rich diet is essential for ensuring adequate fluid intake. A fluid-rich diet includes foods with a high fluid content such as soup, pudding, popsicles, and fruit. A diet history is essential in determining times at which a child receives fluid in the day and to find times when more can be added.

Table 2.12 Estimation of Fluid Requirements According to the Holliday–Segar Method

Body Weight, kg	Maintenance Fluid Requirements
0–10	100 mL/kg
10–20	1,000 mL + 50 mL per kg > 10 kg
> 20	1,500 mL + 20 mL per kg > 20 kg

Example: 18–kg child:

Total maintenance fluid per 24 hours = 1,000 mL + (50 mL × 8 kg)
= 1,400 mL

Source: Data are from reference 6.

Fiber Needs

To calculate fiber needs, it may be helpful to use the DRIs for children. Table 2.13 lists the DRIs for total fiber intake by age (9). Another common method to determine fiber needs is the "age + 5 grams" rule. High fiber foods include whole grains, fruits, and vegetables. The use of commercial fiber supplements may aid in meeting estimated fiber needs.

Table 2.13   Adequate Intakes for Total Fiber

Age	Males, g/d	Females, g/d
0–6 mo	ND	ND
7–12 mo	ND	ND
1–3 y	19	19
4–8 y	25	25
9–13 y	31	26
14–18 y	38	26

Abbreviation: ND, not determined.
Source: Data are from reference 9.

NUTRITION ASSESSMENT OF MEDICATION USE AND POTENTIAL DRUG-NUTRIENT INTERACTIONS

Side effects of certain medications can affect appetite, food intake, and growth. Timing of medication and whether the medication should be taken with foods or liquids is important information and can affect the medication's usefulness. Some medications can cause digestive problems such as constipation or diarrhea; other medications can deplete nutrients from the body. The long-term use of any medication and the use of multiple medications should be noted in the nutrition assessment, and comments about the consequences documented. Box 2.15 lists some of the most common drug-nutrient interactions of medications used with several chronic conditions of children with special health care needs (2,11,12).

Box 2.15   Drug–Nutrient Interactions

Antibiotics
- Nutrients affected: Minerals, fats, protein.
- Overall effect: Temporary decrease in absorption (resulting from diarrhea, nausea, and/or vomiting); destroys "good" intestinal bacteria flora.
- Prevention: Acidophilus and other probiotics may counteract loss of intestinal flora.

Anticonvulsants
- Nutrients affected: vitamins D, K, B-6, and B-12; folate, calcium.
- Overall effect: Decrease nutrient absorption or stores.
- Prevention: Recommend diet high in these nutrients. Vitamin and mineral supplements may be appropriate; seek physician approval as supplementation may influence drug effectiveness.

Cardiac Medications (Diuretics)
- Nutrients affected: Potassium, magnesium, calcium, folate.
- Overall effect: Loss or depletion of nutrient stores; some diuretics can produce these effects; may also cause nausea, diarrhea, and vomiting that lead to reduced food intake.
- Prevention: Recommend foods and fluids high in potassium and magnesium. Suggest strategies to help with decreased appetite.

Corticosteroids
- Used with asthma, arthritis, gastrointestinal disease, cardiac disease, cancer, muscular dystrophy, etc.
- Nutrients affected: Calcium, phosphorus, glucose, vitamin D, protein, sodium, water, zinc, vitamin C, potassium.

(continued)

Box 2.15   Drug–Nutrient Interactions (continued)

Corticosteroids (continued)
- Overall effect: Long–term use can cause stunting of growth; can deplete calcium and phosphorus that can result in bone loss; can affect glucose levels. May also increase appetite, leading to weight gain. Also can cause fluid retention and require monitoring of sodium. Can cause peptic disease, vomiting/diarrhea.
- Prevention: Monitor weight, laboratory values. Supplement with calcium and vitamin D.

Laxative/Bulk Agents
- Nutrients affected: Fat–soluble vitamins.
- Overall effect: Some are bulking agents and others are laxatives. Some laxatives may deplete fat–soluble vitamins when used long–term.
- Prevention: Encourage a diet high in fiber and fluid to wean child off medication. Regimen may need to be altered if a child changes the amount of fiber or fluid they take. Check with physician for alternative medication that will not deplete stores. Encourage weight bearing exercise.

Anti–GERD Medications
- Nutrients affected: Vitamin B-12, iron, calcium.
- Overall effect: Long–term loss of iron, vitamin B-12, and calcium. May cause nausea and diarrhea.
- Prevention: Diet high in these nutrients; monitor laboratory values.

Stimulants
- Used for attention deficit/hyperactivity disorder.
- Overall effect: Can decrease appetite, cause weight loss; may affect overall growth.
- Prevention: Have child eat before each medication dosage if possible. Choose meals at which they are most hungry and encourage larger amounts of intake at those times. Monitor growth and discuss with physician if it is affected.

(continued)

Box 2.15 Drug–Nutrient Interactions (continued)

Sulfonamides
- Used in spina bifida.
- Nutrients affected: Vitamin C, protein, folate, iron.
- Overall effect: Promotes crystallization of large doses of vitamin C in the bladder; inhibits protein synthesis; decreases serum folate and iron.
- Prevention: Avoid supplementation of vitamin C in large doses (>1,000 mg). Increase intake of high–folate foods. Unable to use color or odor of urine as a determinant of hydration status.

Tranquilizers
- Overall effect: Increases appetite; results in excessive weight gain.
- Prevention: Recommend a low–calorie diet, if appropriate. Monitor weight.

Antipsychotics
- Nutrients affected: Sodium, potassium.
- Overall effect: Decreases nutrient absorption. Increases weight gain.
- Prevention: Monitor weight and laboratory test values.

Source: Data are from references 2, 11, and 12.

NUTRITION ASSESSMENT OF USE OF COMPLEMENTARY/ALTERNATIVE MEDICINE

Similar to prescription and over-the counter medications, forms of complementary and alternative medicine (CAM) can have nutritional consequences, and the nutrition assessment should include any use of CAM (see Table 2.14) (13).

Table 2.14   Nutrition Assessment of Patients Who May Use Complementary or Alternative Nutrition Therapy: Documentation Guidelines

Area of Nutrition Assessment	Reasons for Concern/Documentation Recommendations
Anthropometric data	Alterations in growth can occur with restricted diets.
Dietary intake	Note any excesses or deficiencies in nutrients and general food categories. Long–term elimination of certain foods groups (such as dairy) without compensations can lead to dietary deficiencies (such as calcium and protein).
Food and plant allergies or intolerances	Patients with known plant allergies may exhibit reactions to herbal products from the same category.
Current intake of supplements	It is important to identify the types of supplements the child is currently taking; documentation should include the dosage, duration of use, who recommended the product, and whether the primary physician is aware of use.
Caregiver's plans for implementation	Make note of the proposed treatment that the caregivers are considering. Document your assessment to the proposed treatment.

Source: Data are from reference 13.

NUTRITION INTERVENTIONS TO MODIFY ENERGY INTAKE

Nutrition intervention strategies to improve the diets of children with special health care needs include altering energy, macronutrient, micronutrient, fiber, and fluid intake to meet the child's specific needs. Modifying energy intake (either increasing or decreasing) is accomplished by altering the child's fluid and food intake. Box 2.16 presents methods to increase calories in foods and fluids using food sources. Before making recommendations, it is essential to evaluate the caregivers' physical, cultural, and financial abilities to achieve these goals. Commercial products are available (see Box 2.17), but these can be both costly and inconvenient for the family. It is important to try other methods first.

Box 2.16   Practical Food Choices to Increase Energy Intake for Children

Protein Foods
- Peanut butter (94 kcal/Tbsp): On bread, toast, crackers, fruit, vegetables, tortillas, baked goods; in milkshakes, hot cereal
- Chopped nuts[a] (50 kcal/Tbsp): In puddings, salads, casseroles, baked goods; on hot cereals, vegetables, fruits, ice cream
- Hummus or bean spread (17 kcal/Tbsp): On bread, crackers, tortillas; as a dip for vegetables; mixed with cheese, potatoes
- Pesto (56 kcal/Tbsp): On pasta, bread, potatoes, sandwiches, pizza

Milk and Dairy Products
- Whole milk (20 kcal/oz): Add to "instant breakfast," hot chocolate, soups, cooked cereals
- Evaporated whole milk (25 kcal/Tbsp): In place of whole milk in desserts, meat dishes, baked goods, milkshakes, soups, and cooked cereals
- Ice cream (~17 kcal/Tbsp; varies): In milkshakes/fruit smoothies; as topping on baked desserts
- Cream, heavy (60 kcal/Tbsp): On cereals, replacement for part of milk in puddings, hot chocolate, milkshakes, baked goods, soups, sauces
- Cream, half and half (20 kcal/Tbsp): On cereals, replacement for part of milk in puddings, hot chocolate, milkshakes, baked goods, soups, sauces

(continued)

**Box 2.16   Practical Food Choices to Increase Energy Intake
for Children** (continued)

- Dry milk powder, instant form (16 kcal/Tbsp)[b]: Add to
  whole milk, milkshakes, casseroles, soups, sauces, gravy,
  meatloaf, egg salad, chicken salad, tuna salad, potatoes,
  macaroni and cheese, pudding, cereals, baked goods
- Cheese (120 kcal/oz): On bread, toast, vegetables, pasta,
  eggs; in salads, dips, sandwiches; mixed into meatloaf,
  meatballs, soups, potatoes, gravies; as a sauce
- Infant cereal (15 kcal/Tbsp): In fruit, yogurt, vegetables
- Wheat germ, ground flax seed, graham cracker crumbs,
  bread crumbs (25–35 kcal/Tbsp): In baked goods, casseroles, cereals; toppings for fruit, ice cream; in pancakes
- Granola (115 kcal/oz): Topping for yogurt, ice cream,
  applesauce; as trail mix

Fats, Oils, and Sweets
- Vegetable oil (110 kcal/Tbsp): In soups, casseroles, veg-
  etables, gravies, cooked cereals, spaghetti sauce
- Margarine/butter (110 kcal/Tbsp): On pancakes, waffles,
  French toast, bread toast, potatoes, pasta, vegetables; in
  baked goods, casseroles
- Sour cream (25 kcal/Tbsp): On vegetables, potatoes; in
  casseroles, in dips
- Cream cheese (50 kcal/Tbsp): On toast, sandwiches, bagels,
  baked goods; in dips, scrambled eggs, baked goods
- Mayonnaise (100 kcal/Tbsp): On sandwiches, pasta; in
  salads, deviled eggs, vegetable dips
- Salad dressing (75–100 kcal/Tbsp); gravy, barbecue sauce,
  ketchup (20–25kcal/Tbsp): On meats, potatoes, pasta,
  vegetables; in casseroles
- Sweetened coconut flakes (25 kcal/Tbsp)
- Avocado (18 kcal/Tbsp): In sandwiches, pasta, salads, dip,
  eggs, vegetables
- Corn syrup (60 kcal/Tbsp): On cereals, fruit; milkshakes,
  milk
- Jams, jellies, syrups, apple butter (40–50 kcal/Tbsp): On
  bread, toast, waffles, pancakes, biscuits, bagels, French toast,
  ice cream, baked goods

(continued)

**Box 2.16   Practical Food Choices to Increase Energy Intake
              for Children** (continued)

- Chocolate syrup, sugar (white brown, powdered), molasses
  (40–50 kcal/Tbsp): On ice cream, cereal, waffles, pancakes;
  in milk drinks, baked goods
- Chocolate chips, rainbow sprinkles (50–75 kcal/Tbsp): On
  ice cream; in waffles, pancakes, baked goods
- Carnation Instant Breakfast (130 kcal/packet): Add to puddings, yogurts, milkshakes, plain whole milk or half and half

---

[a]Do not offer to children younger than 4 years or those who have oral–motor delays
because of the risk of choking.
[b]Too much nonfat dry milk should not be added to foods for children younger than
2 years or children with medically complex conditions because it may result in an
overload of protein on the kidneys. Check with the physician before recommending
this additive.

**Box 2.17   Commercial Modulars to Increase Energy Intake
              for Children**[a]

Amino acids: Essential amino acid mix (28.44 kcal/Tbsp)

Carbohydrate
- Polycal (29 kcal/Tbsp)
- Polycose (23 kcal/Tbsp)

Protein
- Beneprotein (4 kcal/Tbsp)
- ProMod (49.5 kcal/Tbsp)
- Protifar (14.92 kcal/Tbsp)

Fat: MCT oil (115 kcal/Tbsp)

Combination
- Benecalorie: protein, fat, and carbohydrate (110 kcal/Tbsp)
- Duocal: carbohydrate and fat (42 kcal/Tbsp)
- MCT Procal: protein, fat, and carbohydrate (105 kcal/sachet
  [16 g])
- Procal: protein, fat, and carbohydrate (100 kcal/sachet
  [15 g])
- Scandishake powder (600 kcal/packet)

---

[a]Always check product labels or Web sites for current information.

FOOD HYPERSENSITIVITIES

Adverse reactions to food, called food allergy or hypersensitivity, and food intolerance, are common worldwide. Approximately 2.5% of populations report food-induced complications, which may be gastrointestinal, respiratory, dermatologic, behavioral, or systemic in nature. The National Institute of Allergy and Infectious Diseases (NIAID) reports data on approximate percent of food allergies in children and adults by specific foods (www.niaid .nih.gov). A food allergy occurs when the immune system reacts adversely to a normally harmless component of a food. The component of the food causing the allergy is called an allergen, which is from a protein component of the food. All other reactions (non–immune mediated), previously referred to as food intolerance, should be referred to as non-allergic food hypersensitivity (14,15). The reactions to both food allergy and non-allergic food hypersensitivity can be similar, but anaphylaxis is exclusive to food allergy. See Box 2.18 for an overview (14,15).

Box 2.18   Overview of Adverse Reactions to Foods

IgE–mediated Hypersensitivity (Allergy)
- *Process:* Presence of food allergen–specific IgE.
- *Diagnosis:* (*a*) Blood tests to identify the presence of food–allergen specific IgE; (*b*) scratch or prick skin tests (these are not routinely carried out with foods because of the high number of false positive and false negative reactions).
- *Management:* Elimination of the identified food allergen.

Eosinophilic Esophagitis/Gastroenteritis/Proctocolitis
- *Process:* Presence of eosinophils in the esophagus (esophagitis); stomach and small intestine (gastroenteritis); or colon (protocolitis).

(continued)

Box 2.18   Overview of Adverse Reactions to Foods (continued)

Eosinophilic Esophagitis/Gastroenteritis/Proctocolitis (continued)
- *Diagnosis:* Biopsy of the affected region; there are no tests to determine the specific foods involved.
- *Management:* Elimination of the foods most frequently associated with the condition diagnosed.

Lactose Intolerance
- *Process:* Lack of the enzyme (lactase) that breaks down lactose into its constituent monosccaharides (glucose and galactose). Undigested lactose passes into the colon where it is fermented, causing the GI symptoms associated with the condition.
- *Diagnosis:* Several tests indicate the condition after consumption of lactose including (*a*) hydrogen breath test; (*b*) glucose and galactose levels in blood; (*c*) reducing substance in stool.
- *Management:* Elimination of lactose from the diet. This does not involve removing all milk products: those free from lactose are tolerated.

Celiac Disease (Gluten–Sensitive Enteropathy)
- *Process:* Damage to the intestinal villi in the small intestine as a result of an immunologically–mediated reaction to gluten in certain foods.
- *Diagnosis:* Tests for the presence of specific IgA: (a) IgA–human tissue transglutaminase (TTG) test; or (b) IgA endomysial antibody (EMA) test; or (c) a combination of both are recommended as screening tests. Confirmation may involve jejunal biopsy positive for villous atrophy.
- *Management:* Strict avoidance of wheat, rye, and barley.

Source: Data are from references 14 and 15.

Immune-Mediated Response

In a food allergy, IgE causes the release of inflammatory chemicals from mast cells and basophils. This reaction is the cause of the classic food allergy symptoms, which affect the skin and the respiratory and gastrointestinal tracts. These reactions can be severe enough to cause anaphylaxis, which can result in death. Anaphylaxis, which can be generalized or systemic, requires immediate treatment with epinephrine. Any food can cause an IgE-mediated allergic reaction, but the most common inducers are milk, peanuts, soy, tree nuts, eggs, wheat, fish, and shellfish, accounting for 90% of all food allergic reactions. Routine diagnostic tools to evaluate IgE-mediated reactions are blood tests such as radio-allergosorbent test (RAST) or skin testing. Fluorescence tests are also being used in labs testing for food-specific IgE-mediated reactions. The gold standard continues to be food elimination with food challenge as there are still no completely accurate laboratory tests (14).

Oral allergy syndrome, also known as pollen-food allergy syndrome, is recognized as an immune-mediated reaction. This type of allergy is present with an IgE-mediated reaction. A pollen-food allergy reaction occurs when plant proteins cross-react with specific antigens, particularly birch, ragweed, and grass pollen. Foods that cross-react with birch pollen are raw potatoes, carrots, celery, apples, pears, hazelnuts, and kiwi. Foods that cross-react with ragweed are fresh melons and bananas. Tomato is a food that cross-reacts with grass pollen. The following symptoms can occur with this cross reaction: itching; tingling and/or swelling of the tongue, lips, mouth, or throat; and occasionally anaphylaxis. A child referred for picky eating should be evaluated for oral-allergy syndrome especially if there is a history of food allergies.

Latex-food allergy syndrome, also known as latex-fruit syndrome, occurs when food antigens cross-react with latex antigens. There are 200 or more proteins found in natural rubber latex, which can bind IgE and cross-react with food antigens including, but not limited to, kiwi, potato, tomato, avocado, chestnut, and banana. Foods most commonly associated with latex allergy are banana, avocado, chestnut, and kiwi. Symptoms of latex food allergy syndrome symptoms include itching, eczema, oral-facial swelling, asthma, gastrointestinal symptoms, and anaphylaxis (15).

A child with eosinophilic gastroenteritis/esophagitis can also have IgE-mediated food allergies. Food protein enteropathy is exclusive to young children, but can persist into school age. The child presents with bloody or non-bloody diarrhea, vomiting, and failure to thrive.

Celiac disease and food protein-induced enterocolitis syndromes are examples of a cell-mediated reaction to food. Celiac disease is caused by intolerance to gluten. Food protein-induced enterocolitis syndromes most commonly include intolerances to milk and soy. The diagnoses for these conditions involve biopsies of the GI tract.

The treatment for food allergies is to eliminate the offending food(s) from the diet. The introduction of solid foods for infants with a family history of allergies of certain foods may be delayed (14). The Food Allergy and Anaphylaxis Network (FAAN) (www.foodallergy.org) is a helpful resource for both professionals and parents, providing educational materials, recipe books, monthly newsletters, and other resources.

Non–immune-Mediated Reactions

The most common non–immune-mediated reaction to a specific food is lactose intolerance. The intolerance generally results from a decline in intestinal lactase, the enzyme that breaks down lactose, but can also be due to a loss of lactase-expressing cells of the small intestinal villi due to viral gastroenteritis, radiation enteritis, Crohn's disease, or untreated celiac disease. Symptoms of lactose intolerance include bloating, flatulence, and diarrhea. Diagnosis of lactose intolerance is made with a hydrogen breath test and treatment will depend on the severity of the intolerance but requires a reduction or elimination of lactose from the diet. Food intolerances can include fructose, gluten, and dietary carbohydrates referred to as FODMAPs (fermentable oligosaccharides disaccharides monosaccharides and polypols). Other non–immune-mediated reactions are food toxicity or food poisoning and result in eating food contaminated by staphylococcal enterotoxin such as E coli or salmonella. Reactions to foods can also occur from foods such as caffeine. Most of these reactions cause symptoms such as headaches, rashes, and respiratory complications but no gastrointestinal problems (14,15).

Nutrition Intervention

Nutrition intervention for both food allergies and food intolerances is the same (see Box 2.19). The food or foods must be eliminated from the diet. Families will need help with the selection of alternative foods to substitute for the foods eliminated to meet energy and nutrient needs. Families will benefit from education in reading food labels to avoid the foods eliminated from the diet. Families also need support to educate other family members, friends, daycare providers, and schools. Safety plans must be developed for the child with life-threatening food allergies.

Box 2.19   General Guidelines for Nutrition Interventions for Food Allergies and Intolerances

- Confirm that the specific allergy or intolerance has been diagnosed and the problematic food and food additives to avoid have been accurately identified.
- Provide nutrition education and resources to identify problematic food(s).
- Encourage families to share information with child–care and school staff.
- Assure that child–care and school staffs have developed safety plans jointly using the Food Allergy and Anaphylaxis Network guidelines.
- Encourage as much variety in food intake as possible.
- Provide appropriate substitute foods to replace the nutrients missing from the restricted foods.
- When adding new foods introduce each food separately in order to determine whether the child can tolerate it, per physician's approval.
- Stress the importance of reading food labels each time the food is purchased to identify all sources of the restricted food.

BREASTFEEDING OF CHILDREN WITH SPECIAL HEALTH CARE NEEDS

Breastfeeding for all infants, including those with special needs, is ideal and should be encouraged. Healthcare organizations that work with mothers and infants recommend breastfeeding and breastmilk for every infant except those with galactosemia, inborn errors of metabolism, or when the mother has HIV/AIDS. Breastfeeding an infant with special needs, especially those with low muscle tone, skeletal anomalies (eg, cleft lip and palate), or other oral-motor challenges, is possible if given the correct support by a Board Certified Lactation Consultant (BCLC). Initial skin to skin contact in the first hour or two after birth is important to allow the infant to receive colostrum, be warmed by the mother, have heart rate and respiration be regulated by the mother's body, and even be colonized with the mother's skin bacteria. Breastfeeding can help the mother bond with her infant because it stimulates oxytocin, which would create an early positive attachment to her child with special needs (16–18).

If an infant is born with a condition that does not allow him or her the initial skin to skin contact with the mother, the mother should be encouraged to express her colostrum and then use her finger or a cotton swab to wipe in and around the infants mouth. This should occur before the infant is sent to the NICU or transported elsewhere. If this process is not possible, the infant should be fed via nutrition support (18).

USE OF COMMERCIAL INFANT FORMULA AND PEDIATRIC NUTRITION PRODUCTS

For children for whom breastmilk is unavailable or who do not tolerate breastmilk, commercial infant formulas are available. A variety of formulas is now available. They vary in composition based on its application and the age of the intended consumer. Some act as oral supplements to a child's diet while others serve as a complete nutritional source, which may be administered through a feeding tube.

Table 2.15 describes the general categories of infant formulas, energy density, indications for use, and general comments (19,20). Choose a formula that best fits the child's medical condition. Further modifications can be made to commercial formulas and breastmilk to alter the nutrients including adding more calories, protein, carbohydrates, or fats. Methods for modification should be recommended and calculated by pediatric dietitians or specialty physicians. These methods are not included in this chapter.

Table 2.15   Classification of Commercial Formulas: Types and Indications for Use

Category (Standard Dilution)	Indications for Use	Comments
Cow's milk infant formula (20 kcal/oz)	Standard formula when not breastfeeding	Meets FDA infant formula standards.
Cow's milk "newborn formula" (20 kcal/oz)	Birth to age 3 mo	Meets FDA infant formula standards, has slightly larger amounts of vitamin D.
Soy–based infant formula (20 kcal/oz)	Infants who cannot tolerate cow's milk protein	Meets FDA infant formula standard; not indicated for the premature infant. Recommendation is to recheck for confirmed milk protein allergy once GI symptoms improve.
Premature infant formula (20, 24, 30 kcal/oz)	Premature, VLBW, or LBW infant, until weighs 1,500 g or age 3–4 mo	Usually short–term use, with transition formulas to regular infant formulas as tolerated; close monitoring.
Transition formula (20 kcal/oz)	Premature or LBW infant >1,500 g	In preparation for hospital discharge. Monitor for growth and feeding tolerance.
Follow–up infant formula (20 kcal/oz)	Age 12–24 mo (as alternative to breastmilk)	Composition varies; some can be used with toddlers; used to "bridge the gap" as solid foods are introduced into the diet. Should only be used in children not meeting nutritional needs with solids.

(continued)

Table 2.15 Classification of Commercial Formulas: Types and Indications for Use (continued)

Category (Standard Dilution)	Indications for Use	Comments
Hypoallergenic infant formula (casein hydrolysate), some are 100% whey such as Good Start products (20 kcal/oz)	Infants with suspected GI tract damage. Intolerance to polymeric formulas.	Etiology of GI problem determines correct product. Formula has no intact protein but contains amino acids and small peptides. Fat sources vary. Some are higher in MCT oil.
Elemental infant formula (amino acid–based) (20 kcal/oz)	Infants with cow's milk protein and soy milk allergy or other intolerances to hypoallergenic formulas.	Also used with infants with growth failure due to GERD and food allergies. Synthetic amino acids are protein source.
Polymeric pediatric formulas (30 kcal/oz)	Children ≥ age 1 y.	For children that are not meeting their nutritional needs by mouth. Complete nutrition product. Usually taste better, are easiest to find in stores and are cheapest.
Hydrolyzed pediatric formula (30 kcal/oz)	Children ≥ age 1 y with intolerance to polymeric formula.	Etiology of GI problem determines correct product. Formula has no intact protein but contains amino acids and small peptides. Fat sources vary some with higher volumes of MCT.
Elemental pediatric formula, amino acid–based (30 kcal/oz)	Children ≥ age 1 y with cow's milk protein and soy milk protein allergies.	Synthetic amino acid or protein source.

(continued)

Table 2.15 Classification of Commercial Formulas: Types and Indications for Use (continued)

Category (Standard Dilution)	Indications for Use	Comments
Specialized pediatric formulas for specific diseases or disorders (30 kcal/oz)	Children ≥ 1 y with chronic GI disorders, renal, pulmonary, diabetes, or metabolic diagnoses.	Due to expense generally intended for temporary use if diagnoses will allow (products for metabolic disorders are used for lifetime, with modifications as the child ages). Protein, fat, and carbohydrate sources vary.
Modular products—protein, carbohydrate, fat (varies with product)	To add calories or nutrients to a standard product.	Modulars are used to add either a singular nutrient or combinations (eg, fat and carbohydrate). It is essential to calculate nutrient distribution to assure balance. Additionally, modular components can displace formula. This must be considered when calculating total volume and mixing instructions. Not complete products.
Electrolyte and rehydration products (minimal)	Infants and children. Used during acute phases of diarrhea	Intended for temporary use during acute illness. Not complete products.
Nutrient–dense polymeric products (45–60 kcal/oz)	Children ≥ age 1 y unable to maintain adequate oral intake from food. Intact protein, fats, carbohydrates, vitamins and minerals can meet all nutrient needs at specific volume.	Many varieties, with flavors, with or without fiber, for oral or non–oral feeding (*see also* Chapter 4).

(continued)

Table 2.15 Classification of Commercial Formulas: Types and Indications for Use (continued)

Category (Standard Dilution)	Indications for Use	Comments
Nutrient–dense hydrolyzed products (45 kcal/oz)	Children ≥ age 1 y unable to maintain adequate oral intake from food.	Smaller peptide products generally with more MCT oil.

Abbreviations: FDA, Food and Drug Administration; GERD gastroesophageal reflux disease; GI: gastrointestinal; LBW, low birth weight; VLBW, very low birth weight.
Source: Data are from reference 19.

Target ages, as they pertain to formulas, include infants (younger than 12 months) and pediatrics (ages 1 to 10 years). Typically, infant products are mixed to be 20 kcal/oz (same energy concentration as breastmilk). Products for toddlers and children are typically 30 kcal/oz. For children older than 10 years of age, review formula requirements on a regular basis to determine whether an adult product better meets the patient's nutritional needs. Some pediatric formulas are approved for use in individuals up to 13 years of age.

Cow's milk is the recommended beverage for toddlers and children. In some cases, special products to replace milk may be required to meet energy and nutrient needs. Milk replacement products are generally higher in calories per ounce than cow's milk (see Table 2.15). These formulas should be used either as a complete medical food when a child is unable to consume adequate portions of food or as a supplement to a limited diet.

The composition of a formula may vary in both quantity and structure of micronutrients and macronutrients. A more specialized formula is indicated based on a child's medical condition, tolerance of macronutrients (protein, fat, carbohydrate), goal renal solute load/osmolarity, and vitamin and mineral needs. Additionally, the feeding route (oral or tube, as well as placement of tube) is an essential consideration. Registered dietitians (RDs) in the community should monitor the family's use of the product. Important items to note in follow-up evaluations include gastrointestinal tolerance, weight changes, actual intake as compared with the recommended plan, family's level of satisfaction with the product, and feeding schedule. Refer to Box 2.20 for clinical tips related to the use of formulas (20), and see Chapter 4 for more information about enteral feedings.

Box 2.20 Clinical Tips: Formula Use

- If a special product is used as the child's sole source of nutrition, it is vital to ensure that the child is meeting the Dietary Reference Intake for all nutrients (protein, energy, vitamins, minerals, dietary fiber, fluid, etc). The volume needed to meet the child's nutrient needs will vary from product to product. This information must be calculated and evaluated to ensure the percent distribution of the major nutrients (carbohydrate, protein, and fat) meets standards. Additional calculations are necessary to determine micronutrient intake. The use of computer programs makes this much easier and efficient.
- To increase the energy density of infant formula, such as making a formula that is 24 kcal/oz, it is advised to refer to the manufacturer's guidelines. Methods and measuring tools vary with manufacturer.
- When making a large volume of formula, it may be easier for the family to measure the formula with household measuring cups or portions of a cup. Make sure the family has these available to them. Check with the manufacturer for the conversion factors (ie, number of scoops to equal a portion of a measuring cup or calories per cup conversions).

(continued)

Box 2.20   Clinical Tips: Formula Use (continued)

- If an infant or child is consuming a specialized product, be sure to determine how the family is paying for the product. Many of these products are very expensive and families may not be able to pay for the product. State or federal programs can often assist families if needed. *See* Chapter 5 for more information on ways to obtain reimbursement for specialized products.

- Some children experience gastrointestinal symptoms after a change in nutrition products, even if the nutrient composition seems to be the same. These may include diarrhea, flatulence, distention, etc. Transition to the new product may involve mixing old and new products or a short–term dilution of the new product. The specialty team or pediatrician needs to be aware of intolerances and help families work through transitions.

- Formula and complete nutritional supplements should be refrigerated after they are opened and used within 24 hours. Bacterial contamination and subsequent gastrointestinal problems can occur with improperly stored formula, both at home and school.

- The American Academy of Pediatrics does not recommend the use of low–iron formulas in infant feeding and recommends that all formulas fed to infants be fortified with iron. To be labeled "with iron," infant formulas must contain at least 6.7 mg iron per liter; most standard infant formulas contain approximately 12 mg iron per liter (20).

- It is important to closely monitor infants and children using specialized formulas or supplements to determine whether the child still requires the product. As children grow, their energy and nutrient needs change and the use of the special product should be reassessed. This may be overlooked by others and is the primary responsibility of the registered dietitian.

VITAMIN AND MINERAL SUPPLEMENTATION

Some families want to use vitamin and/or mineral supplements even when they are not necessary (eg, when the child has an adequate intake or is receiving a complete nutrition supplement). Parents may ask about the use of a vitamin and/or mineral supplement as an "insurance policy." If the child is eating a variety of foods from all of the major food groups, is growing well, and is in overall good health, there is no need for a supplement. A standard multivitamin is acceptable if there is suspicion that a patient is not meeting micronutrient needs. Occasionally a patient will require additional supplements in the form of vitamin D, calcium, or fluoride if a diet recall and/or labs indicate deficiency (refer to Table 2.16) (21). When evaluating a patient for potential supplementation needs, it is important to consider not only the diet but also medications with potential for nutrient interactions.

Table 2.16   Indications for Recommending a Pediatric Vitamin and Mineral Supplement

Condition	Reason
Underweight child with chronic low food intake	Low intake of foods to meet nutrient needs.
Child with multiple food allergies	Omission of food groups where nutrients from this food group would typically be obtained.
Tube–fed older child with very low energy intake	Low volume due to low energy requirements may limit vitamins and mineral intake.
Child on medications that alter absorption or utilization of certain nutrients	Nutrient deficiencies due to drug–nutrient interactions.

(continued)

**Table 2.16   Indications for Recommending a Pediatric
Vitamin and Mineral Supplement** (continued)

Condition	Reason
Child with very limited food choices (child with autism, pervasive developmental disorder)	Omission of foods from a food group that provide key nutrients. Often difficult to add a vitamin/mineral supplement because the child may refuse the new item to the diet.

Source: Data are from reference 21.

Generally, the best recommendation is a complete pediatric multivitamin/mineral supplement that meets 100% of the DRIs. The issues of cost, refusal to accept such supplements due to taste, or possible gastrointestinal symptoms should also be discussed with the caregiver. Sometimes families are able to give the supplement at less than the recommended dose, such as every other day, or only half a tablet, and this may be sufficient.

The DRIs include ULs for many nutrients, based on the potential to cause adverse effects at high levels. This is most often of concern when the high levels of nutrients come from supplements. Cumulative nutrient intake from all sources (food, pediatric formulas, and vitamin/mineral supplements) should be compared with the ULs and appropriate recommendations given to the family to assure safety. See Box 2.21 for additional clinical tips (13,16).

Box 2.21   Clinical Tips: Micronutrient Supplementation

- It is helpful for parents to have their child's vitamin or mineral intake assessed by using a diet analysis computer program, based on a recent 2– or 3–day food record.

(continued)

Box 2.21 Clinical Tips: Micronutrient Supplementation
(continued)

- Fluoride is recommended for infants and children who do not have access to fluoride in their water supply (ie, families that have well water, have a water supply that is not fluoridated, or use bottled water). Ready-to-feed infant formulas have fluoride added.
- The American Academy of Pediatrics recommends that exclusively breastfed infants should receive a supplement to ensure an intake of 400 IU of vitamin D per day. Supplementation should begin within the first 2 months of life (16). Supplementation with iron is also recommended but only after 2 months.
- Calcium, iron, vitamin C, and other nutrients that have been reported to be low in diets of healthy children are also likely to be low in children with chronic conditions.
- Families with children with chronic illnesses are more vulnerable to claims from alternative or complementary medicine therapies than other families. If the caregiver is considering the use of a complementary or alternative nutritional therapy for the child, the registered dietitian should document this information in the medical record. Table 2.14 lists information that should be included in the report (13). Many of these products lack sufficient evidence as a treatment mode. Health professionals can collaborate with families to identify if the product or therapy is safe to use in children; whether there are any documented reports on effectiveness of the treatment; potential side effects, and the cost, time, and energy required to provide the therapy.

CASE STUDY 1: GIRL, AGE 5 YEARS, WITH CEREBRAL PALSY

Nutrition Assessment

- Client history: Samantha is a 5-year-old girl with spastic quadriplegic cerebral palsy. Patient presents with minimal weight gain over the last 12 months.
- Biochemical data, medical tests, and procedures: Modified barium swallow indicated patient safe to consume thickened liquids to a nectar consistency without aspiration.
- Medications: Enemas.
- Drug-nutrient interactions: None.
- Multivitamin/mineral supplement: None.
- Anthropometric measurements:
  - Height/length: 102 cm (10th percentile, CDC growth chart).
  - Weight: 14.9 kg (5th percentile, CDC growth chart).
  - BMI: 14.3 (20th percentile, CDC growth chart).
  - Triceps skinfold: 6 mm (5th percentile)—*should be closely monitored for weight loss and or decrease in fat stores.*
- Food and nutrition history:
  - Energy needs: 868 kcal/d (789 kcal/d × 1.1); REE based on Schofield equation (58 kcal/kg/d).
  - Energy intake: 700 kcal/d (47 kcal/kg/d).
  - Protein needs: 15 g/d (1.0 g/kg/d).
  - Protein intake: 15 g/d (1.0 g/kg/d).
  - Fluid needs: 1,245 mL/d.
  - Fluid intake: 1,000 mL/d.
  - Based on 3-day dietary recall the patient's energy intake is 700 kcal/d and protein intake is 15 g/d.

Parents describe feeding as very difficult because their daughter fatigues quickly during the meal.

- Offered soft mashed foods and it takes typically 1 hour to feed a meal. She is not able to self-feed.
- Patient has difficulty staying positioned correctly and often falls asleep during her meal. Liquids are thickened to nectar consistency using rice cereal.
- Commercial nutrition supplements and thickeners have been recommended in the past but are too expensive for the family to purchase.

Nutrition Diagnoses

- Suboptimal oral intake (problem) related to feeding difficulties (etiology) as evidenced by inadequate energy intake based on 3-day food diary as compared to standards and minimal weight gain over the last year (signs and symptoms).
- Suboptimal fluid intake (problem) related to feeding difficulties (etiology) as evidenced by chronic constipation—1 hard stool every 3 days; fluid intake falls short of estimated maintenance needs by 245 mL/d (signs and symptoms).
- Limited access to food (problem) related to family's financial constraints (etiology) as evidenced by inability to purchase commercial thickeners and/or supplements (signs and symptoms).
- Chewing difficulty (problem) related to oral motor difficulties secondary to cerebral palsy (etiology) as evidenced by lengthy feedings, inability to meet calorie and fluid needs (signs and symptoms).
- Swallowing difficulty (problem) related to poor motor control secondary to cerebral palsy (etiology) as evidenced by lengthy feedings, inability to meet calorie and fluid needs (signs and symptoms).

Nutrition Intervention

- Nutrition prescription:
  - 870 kcal/d diet with nectar thick liquids.
  - Maintenance fluid needs: 1,245 mL/d.
- Nutrition interventions:
  - Add ½ to 1 tablespoon of ground flaxseed, butter, sun butter, nut butter, or other nutrient dense foods 2 or 3 times a day to soft foods to increase calories by 170 per day and promote weight gain.
  - Increase fluids by 8 oz/d to meet estimated fluid requirements, using a nectar consistency. Be sure to consult with feeding and swallowing specialist regarding thickeners and methods to achieve nectar consistency.
  - Secure financial assistance through social worker at area agency to coordinate access to thickeners for beverages and liquid supplement. If the feeding specialist approves of a less expensive thickener such as infant cereal, this may be used instead of the more expensive thickeners.
  - If and when supplements are available the goal would be up to 8 oz/d.
  - Referral to feeding specialist for assistance in chewing and swallowing difficulties.

Nutrition Monitoring/Evaluation

- Weight: achieve BMI between the 10th and 25th percentiles.
- Output: Goal of 1 soft bowel movement daily.
- Fluid intake and adherence to the use of supplements/thickeners with all fluids as confirmed by feeding specialist.
- Follow up 1 month.

CASE STUDY 2: BOY, AGE 5 YEARS, WITH AUTISM

Nutrition Assessment

- Client history: Ralph is a 5-year-old boy with autism, anemia, low tone, and obesity.
- Biochemical data, medical tests, and procedures: Hemoglobin 9.5mg/dL.
- Medications: Risperdal.
- Drug-nutrient interactions: Increased appetite, increased weight, obesity.
- Multivitamin/Mineral Supplement: None.
- Anthropometric measurements
  - Height: 109.2 cm (50th percentile CDC growth chart).
  - Weight: 23.7 kg (95th percentile CDC growth chart).
  - BMI: 19.9 (> 95th percentile CDC growth chart).
- Food and nutrition history:
  - Energy needs: 1,226 kcal/d (REE = 1,021 kcal/d × 1.2 by Schofield).
  - Energy intake: 1,800 kcal/d.
  - Protein needs: 26 g/d (1.1 g/kg/d).
  - Protein intake: 35 g/d (1.5 g/kg/d).
  - Fluid needs: 1,574 mL/d.
  - Fluid intake: 1,200 mL/d.
  - Patient will only eat corn chips, bagels, French fries, grapes, and chicken nuggets. He refuses to eat any vegetables or red meat. He prefers salty and crunchy foods and foods that are beige in color, and drinks approximately 40 oz whole milk per day through a bottle.

Nutrition Diagnoses

- Excessive energy intake (problem) related to drug-nutrient interaction, low tone, and poor food choices (etiology) as evidenced by BMI greater than 95th percentile (signs and symptoms).
- Suboptimal micronutrient intake (problem) related to highly restrictive diet (etiology) as evidenced by not meeting DRIs for iron, zinc, fiber, vitamin C, and fluids (signs and symptoms).

Nutrition Intervention

- Nutrition prescription: 1,200 kcal/d balanced diet, or adjusted as needed, to promote gradual decrease in BMI to less than the 95th percentile.
- Nutrition interventions:
  - Decrease milk consumption to 24 to 32 oz of low-fat milk.
  - Refer to feeding therapist with goals of increasing dietary variety.
  - Instruction on iron-rich diet and recommendation of multivitamin supplement with iron. Will consult with feeding therapist as to the best method to provide supplement.
  - Recommend obtaining laboratory tests for iron status and lipid profile.
  - Increase intake of foods from all food groups and encourage dietary variety.

Nutrition Monitoring/Evaluation

- Weight: promote weight loss of 1 to 2 pounds per month, or at least weight maintenance, while linear growth continues in order to achieve a gradual decrease in BMI to within the 50th and 85th percentiles.

- Compare dietary intake based on 24-hour recall to standards for age.
- Assess available laboratory values.
- Follow up in 1 month.

CASE STUDY 3: BOY, AGE 15 MONTHS, WITH MULTIPLE FOOD ALLERGIES AND ASTHMA

Nutrition Assessment

- Client history: George is a 15-month-old boy with food allergies to dairy, soy, wheat, eggs, and peanuts; failure to thrive; and asthma. Weight and height percentiles dropped from the 50th percentile to below the 3rd percentile from age 6 months to age 15 months.
- Biochemical data, medical tests, and procedures: CAP RAST blood test positive for dairy, soy, wheat, eggs, and peanuts.
- Physical findings: Often irritable and wakes frequently during the night.
- Medications: Albuterol—inhaled as needed.
- Drug-nutrient interactions: None.
- Multivitamin/mineral supplement: hypoallergenic pediatric chewable or liquid multivitamin/mineral supplement.
- Anthropometric measurements:
  - Length: 71 cm (<3rd percentile CDC growth chart).
  - Weight: 7.5 kg (<3rd percentile CDC growth chart).
  - Weight/height: IBW 8.6 kg (<3rd percentile CDC growth chart).
  - Triceps skinfold: 5 mm (<5th percentile).
  - Subscapular skinfold: 3 mm (<5th percentile).

- Food and nutrition history:
  - Energy needs: 878 kcal/d (117 kcal/kg/d for catch-up growth).
  - Energy intake: 700 kcal/d (93 kcal/kg/d).
  - Protein needs: 9 g/d (1.2 g/kg/d).
  - Protein intake: 6 g/d (0.8 g/kg/d).
  - Fluid needs: 750 mL/d.
  - Fluid intake: 650 mL/d.
  - 24-hour diet recall reveals child's diet is low in energy, protein, iron, calcium, and zinc.
  - Mother reports son will only eat rice cakes, rice puffs, chicken, and applesauce. He will only drink rice milk in small amounts and water. When offered new foods he usually will take one bite and then spit the food out.

Nutrition Diagnosis

Suboptimal energy intake (problem) related to multiple food allergies and self-restricted diet (etiology) as evidenced by not meeting estimated needs for energy, protein, iron, calcium and zinc (signs and symptoms).

Nutrition Intervention

- Nutrition prescription: 110–120 kcal/kg/d diet that is free of wheat, dairy, soy, egg and peanuts.
- Nutrition intervention:
  - High calorie diet; wheat-, dairy-, soy-, egg- and peanut-free diet instructed.
  - Samples provided for pediatric elemental formula. Instructed family on how to mix with fortified rice milk, Tang, or Kool-aid for better flavor. (Make sure family uses fortified rice milk; he may benefit from a product such as Elecare or Neocate Jr. to meet his nutritional needs.)

○ Provide food allergy resources. Refer to Food Allergy and Anaphylaxis Network (FAAN).
○ Referral to feeding therapy for helping with acceptance of new foods.

Nutrition Monitoring/Evaluation

- Weight: achieve weight-for-stature greater than 5th percentile.
- Intake: Compare 24-hour recall to standards to ensure nutrition adequacy on restricted diet.
- Check parent understanding and compliance with nutrition instruction of restricted diet.

REFERENCES

1. Ekvall SW, Ekvall VK. *Pediatric Nutrition in Chronic Diseases and Developmental Disorders.* 2nd ed. New York, NY: Oxford University Press; 2005.
2. Nardella M, Campo L, Ogata B, eds. *Nutrition Interventions for Children with Special Health Care Needs.* Olympia, WA: Washington State Department of Health; 2002.
3. Position of the American Dietetic Association: providing nutrition services for infants, children and adults with developmental disabilities and special health care needs. *J Am Diet Assoc.* 2004; 104:97–107.
4. Samour PQ, King K. *Handbook of Pediatric Nutrition.* 3rd ed. Sudbury, MA: Jones Bartlett Publishers; 2005.
5. Herr SM. *Herb-Drug Interaction Handbook.* 2nd ed. Nassau, NY: Church Street Books; 2002.
6. Hendricks KM, Duggan C. *Manual of Pediatric Nutrition.* 4th ed. Hamilton, ON: BC Decker; 2005.
7. Feeding the child. In: Kleinman RE, ed. *Pediatric Nutrition Handbook.* 5th ed. Elk Grove Village, IL: American Academy of Pediatrics; 2004:119–136.
8. American Academy of Pediatrics Committee on Nutrition. The use and misuse of fruit juice in pediatrics. *Pediatrics.* 2001;107: 1210–1213.

9. Institute of Medicine. *Dietary Reference Intakes: The Essential Guide to Nutrient Requirements.* Washington, DC: National Academies Press; 2006.

10. Murray P, Lansing G, Weston S. Enteral management of children with special health care needs. *Nutr Focus.* 2006;21(4): 1–8.

11. Nutrition management of seizure disorders. In: Nevin-Folino N, ed. *Pediatric Manual of Clinical Dietetics.* 2nd ed. Chicago, IL: American Dietetic Association; 2003:423–450.

12. Pronsky ZM. *Food-Medication Interactions.* 14th ed. Birchrunville, PA: Food-Medication Interactions; 2006.

13. Holland M. Communicating with families concerning the use of complementary or alternative nutritional therapies. *Building Block for Life.* 2000;24:6–11.

14. Food hypersensitivity. In: Kleinman RE, ed. *Pediatric Nutrition Handbook.* 5th ed. Elk Grove Village, IL: American Academy of Pediatrics; 2004:593–607.

15. Mahr TA. Food allergy diagnosis: your questions answered. *Food Allergy News.* 2009;18(3):1,9.

16. American Academy of Pediatrics. Policy statement. Breastfeeding and the use of human milk. *Pediatrics.* 2005;115: 496–506.

17. Thomas J, Marinelli KA, Hennessy M; Academy of Breastfeeding Medicine Protocol Committee. ABM Protocol #16: breastfeeding the hypotonic infant. *Breastfeed Med.* 2007; 2:112–118.

18. Ludington-Hoe S. *Kangaroo Care: The Best You Can Do to Help Your Preterm Infant.* New York, NY: Bantam; 1993.

19. Hattner JT. Pediatric Formula Update 2006. *Nutr Focus.* 2006;20(6):1–11.

20. American Academy of Pediatrics, Committee on Nutrition. Iron-fortified infant formulas. *Pediatrics.* 1999;104: 119–123.

21. Vitamins. In: Kleinman RE, ed. *Pediatric Nutrition Handbook.* 5th ed. Elk Grove Village, IL: American Academy of Pediatrics; 2004:339–365.

Chapter 3

Feeding and Eating

Aaron Owens, MS, RD, CSP, CD

INTRODUCTION TO FEEDING AND EATING

The nutritional health of an infant or child is determined by adequate consumption of either food or other nutritional products. Development of feeding behavior depends on the maturation of the central nervous system, which controls the acquisition of fine, gross, and oral-motor skills. Each of these skills influences the child's ability to consume food (1). Feeding and swallowing skill acquisition is critical to infants and young children as they develop self-regulation that eventually leads to independent feeding (2).

Typical development of feeding skills proceeds in an orderly and predictable sequence (see Box 3.1) (1,3,4). Foods should be introduced to match the developmental skill level of the child. The growth and development for all oral skills is believed to continue until approximately 3 years of age, when the typically developing child should have obtained all the basic oral skills needed as an adult (1,4). Understanding normal oral-motor development is essential for assessing children who may be at risk for feeding problems. Presence of feeding difficulties and/or delays can have a significant impact on a child's overall nutrition and hydration status. Delays in introduction to a variety of food textures can also have a detrimental impact on speech development (5). Assessment of physical, psychological, and developmental readiness is essential when advancing from a liquid to solid food diet.

Box 3.1 Typical Development of Feeding Skills

Birth to Age 4 Months
- Oral motor skills: Rooting, sucking, swallowing and extrusion reflexes; head control initiated; tongue protrudes, mouth opens in anticipation.
- Self-feeding skills: Begins to reach for objects.
- Types of food: Breastmilk, infant formula.

Ages 4 to 6 Months
- Oral motor skills: Voluntary sucking begins; disappearance of extrusion reflex; transfers food from front to back of tongue; purses and smacks lips; more mature trunk control.
- Self-feeding skills: Recognizes breast/bottle; able to grasp objects (bottle) voluntarily; mouths objects.
- Types of food: Infant cereal, strained fruit/vegetables.

Ages 6 to 8 Months
- Oral motor skills: Closes lips around spoon; vertical chewing begins; tongue lateralization emerges; munching continues.
- Self-feeding skills: Able to sit alone (ready for high chair); begins to hold bottle independently; plays with spoon; brings food to mouth; begins to sip from cup; voluntary release and resecure of hand-held objects.
- Types of food: Infant cereal; strained to junior texture of fruits, vegetables and meats; add large, soft finger foods; juice/formula from a cup.

Ages 8 to 10 Months
- Oral motor skills: Voluntary bite emerges; tongue begins to move independently from jaw; transfers food from center to sides of mouth.

(continued)

Box 3.1   Typical Development of Feeding Skills (continued)

Ages 8 to 10 Months (continued)
- Self-feeding skills: Finger feed with palmar grasp; holds own bottle without help; sips from a cup without spilling; decreased fluid intake as solids increase; coordinates hand-to-mouth movement.
- Types of food: Decrease use of strained foods; add finely chopped or mashed table foods; juice/formula in a cup.

Ages 10 to 12 Months
- Oral motor skills: Rotary chewing begins; licks food from lower lip; tooth eruption; improved ability to bite and chew; holds cup without help; finger feed with pincer grasp; bites food.
- Self-feeding skills: Begins self-feeding with a spoon.
- Types of food: Soft, chopped table foods; small finger foods.

Ages 12 to 18 Months
- Oral motor skills: Takes 4 to 5 continuous swallows of liquid; improved rotary chewing.
- Self-feeding skills: Drinking from a cup at all meals; practice with spoon improves.
- Types of foods: Progression of textured table food continues; begin to wean from bottle; more cup drinking.

Ages 18 to 36 Months
- Oral motor skills: Development of all oral movements needed for eating, except refined rotary jaw movement.
- Self-feeding skills: More practice and maturity with skills.
- Types of foods: Regular table foods; weaned from bottle; liquids in a cup; take caution with foods that may cause choking.

Age > 36 Months
- All basic oral skills needed as an adult are present.

Source: Data are from references 1, 3, and 4.

Physical Readiness for Solids

Initial resistance to spoon-feeding is common, and gag reflex of varying degrees is apparent until the infant is about 7 to 9 months of age. Choking, despite the chronological age, indicates infant is not ready to advance to solid foods. When introducing foods, feed one food for 7 to 10 days and watch for any symptoms of intolerance, such as skin rashes, vomiting, wheezing, or diarrhea (3).

Psychological Readiness for Solids

By 6 months, an infant is able to indicate desire for food by opening his/her mouth, leaning forward to indicate hunger, and leaning back or turning away to communicate disinterest or satiety. Until the infant can communicate these cues, feeding of solids will likely represent a type of force feeding, potentially leading to overfeeding and/or obesity. Infant should be given independence in regards to controlling the timing of feeds in an effort to promote self-regulation of hunger and satiety (3). Children breastfed for at least 6 months have been reported to be less likely to be picky eaters as they have been exposed to multiple flavors in the mother's diet that pass through breastmilk (2).

Matching Feeding Advancement with Developmental Milestones

The goal of feeding advancement is to transition from a liquid diet to a well-balanced table food diet, while encouraging development of age appropriate feeding skills. Any of the following oral-motor activity components listed below may be negatively affected by a child's overriding medical condition:

- Body positioning
- Fine and gross motor skills

- Social interactions
- Cognitive level

Children with developmental delays may show slow progression in their development of eating skills. The ability of the child, not the chronological age, should dictate the oral feeding stage. Encouraging parents to be their child's best advocate should begin early.

FEEDING BEHAVIORS

Feeding is an important element of parent–child relations beginning in infancy and continuing through adolescence. Behavioral problems are more common in children with special health care needs and chronic illnesses because the parent and child may be struggling with control and communication difficulties. The key to successful intervention is to separate food-related behavior and parent–child behavior. Parents may misinterpret an oral-motor problem as "bad" behavior or lack of appetite, rather than recognizing that the child may not be developmentally ready for a specific food or texture. Box 3.2 outlines distinguishing features of picky eaters vs problem feeders, and Table 3.1 (6) describes appropriate infant–caregiver feeding interactions. Successful eating is not only dependent upon the parent–child interaction, but the parent and/or child's ability to recognize and interpret hunger and satiety cues.

Box 3.2   Picky Eaters vs Problem Feeders

Picky Eaters
- Decreased range or variety of foods consumed to fewer than 30 or more foods.
- Foods lost due to "burn out" resulting from a food jag are usually regained after a 2-week break.

(continued)

Box 3.2   Picky Eaters vs Problem Feeders (continued)

Picky Eaters (continued)
- New foods are usually tolerated on a plate and can be touched or tasted (even if reluctantly).

Problem Feeders
- Restricted range or variety of foods including typically less than 20 different foods.
- Foods lost due to food jags are *not* reacquired.
- Cries and "falls apart" when presented with new foods.

Source: Adapted with permission from Kay Toomey, PhD.

Table 3.1   Infant–Caregiver Feeding Interactions

Infant Action	Caregiver Response
Cries or whimpers	Initiate feeding
Opens mouth in anticipation; smacks lips after each spoonful	Continue feeding
Turns head away from spoon; averts eyes; pushes spoon away	Stop feeding

Source: Data are from reference 7.

Appetite and Eating Behavior Distortions

Children with developmental delays give cues to caregivers about hunger and fullness, but they may be subtle and nonverbal. If positive response to hunger cue is not received, the child may stop attempting to give signals of hunger and underfeeding may result (1,7).

Caregivers who give food to satisfy all types of discomforts may lead to the child's inability to discriminate hunger from other discomforts. Some children may have a distorted sense of hunger and satiety as a result of their medical or developmental condition (see Box 3.3 for a list of satiety cues) (1,6). An infant with distorted hunger cues may require the parent(s) to wake the infant on a schedule; at least until the hunger sensation develops (1,7).

Box 3.3   Satiety Cues

• Draws head away from the nipple
• Fusses or cries during feeding
• Averts gaze away from feeding
• Blocks mouth with hands
• Changes posture
• Keeps mouth tightly closed
• Shakes head as if to say "no"
• Hands become more active
• Sputters with tongue and lips
• Falls asleep

Source: Data are from references 1 and 6.

When a caregiver is anxious about a child's food intake, it is common for children to use negative food-related behaviors as a way to manipulate and gain control. See Box 3.4 for a list of positive and negative feeding behaviors (7).

Box 3.4   Positive vs Negative Feeding Behaviors

Positive Feeding Behaviors
• Acceptance of a wide variety of foods and textures
• Self-feeding at an appropriate developmental level
• Remaining seated during mealtime
• Eating at a moderate pace
• Eating and drinking quietly
• Using utensils appropriately
• Chewing and swallowing with the mouth closed
<div align="right">(continued)</div>

Box 3.4   Positive vs Negative Feeding Behaviors (continued)

Negative Feeding Behaviors
- Crying when food is offered
- Refusal to accept food
- Throwing food
- Gagging and vomiting in response to food offered
- Inability or unwillingness to sit still during mealtime

Source: Data are from reference 7.

FEEDING PROBLEMS: OVERVIEW

Feeding problems are defined as the inability or refusal to eat certain foods due to sensory processing/integration issues, obstructive lesions, or psychological factors and may occur in up to 25% to 35% of infants and children (3). A child who requires more than 30 to 40 minutes to feed on a regular basis is considered to have a feeding problem (2). Assessment should be as comprehensive as possible to determine the causes and extent of the problem. Effective interventions can then be implemented. Box 3.5 lists physical, behavioral/emotional, and environmental factors that may lead to a child's refusal to eat.

Box 3.5   Reasons Children Will Not Eat (Aversive Conditioning)

Physical Factors
- Pain:
  - Reflux
  - Vomiting
  - Retching/gagging
  - Esophagitis/sore throat
  - Acute illness
  - Colitis/stomach pain
  - Infectious conditions

(continued)

Box 3.5   Reasons Children Will Not Eat (Aversive Conditioning)
(continued)

- Malaise/discomfort:
  - Nausea
  - Nervous system arousal
  - Allergies
  - Cardiac condition
  - Fatigue
  - Constipation
  - Stomach distention
  - Congestion
  - Renal conditions
- Immature motor, oral-motor, and swallowing skills:
  - Choking/overstuffing
  - Immature chew and/or tongue coordination
  - Aspiration
  - Oral processing problems
  - Breathing difficulties
  - Balance problems/instability
  - Oral hypersensitivity
  - Poor hand-to-mouth coordination

Behavioral/Emotional Factors
- Child factors:
  - Difficult temperament
  - Highly distractible
  - Low frustration tolerance
  - Neophobic
  - Hyperactive
  - Anxious and/or fearful
  - Depression
  - Lack of responsiveness to internal hunger cues
  - Texture hypersensitivity
  - Oral aversion
  - Information and/or sensory processing problems
- Parent factors:
  - Does not provide positive reinforcement
  - Provides poor modeling of appropriate eating behaviors

(continued)

Box 3.5   Reasons Children Will Not Eat (Aversive Conditioning)
(continued)

- ○ Models poor eating behaviors and/or personal dislikes
- ○ Restricts diet due to fears of child getting fat
- ○ Overfeeds/force feeds due to distorted vision of normal weight
- ○ Focuses primarily on weight gain vs. interaction
- ○ Has extreme fears about lack of weight gain
- ○ Has inappropriate developmental expectations
- ○ Does not set clear limits on child because of fears and/or guilt about medical/emotional fragility of the child
- ○ Punishes the child at meals
- ○ Provides non-contingent parenting
- ○ Coerces child
- ○ Distracts child
- ○ Repetitively interrupts feeding
- ○ Provides inconsistent parenting

Environmental Factors
- Lack of exposure to food
- Allowed to graze all day
- No exposure to "normal" meal
- Food insecurity
- Lack of structure to meals
- Overstimulating household
- Toys/television/games during meals

Source: Adapted with permission from Kay Toomey, PhD.

Children with feeding problems are unlikely to "out-grow" abnormal feeding behaviors without interventions. Some children find the work of eating more fatiguing than drinking. Thus, inadequate intake of nutrients to support appropriate growth and development may result in failure to thrive. If oral skills are not sufficient, a complete nutritional drink may be needed in place of meals (7).

COMMON ORAL-MOTOR FEEDING PROBLEMS

The following are common oral-motor feeding issues
(1,7):

- **Tonic bite reflex**: strong, involuntary jaw closure
  when teeth and gums are stimulated
- **Tongue thrust**: forceful and repetitive protrusion of
  an often bunched or thickened tongue in response to
  oral stimulation
- **Jaw thrust**: forceful opening of the jaw to the maxi-
  mal extent during eating, drinking, attempts to speak,
  or general excitement
- **Tongue retraction**: pulling back the tongue within
  the oral cavity on the presentation of food, spoon,
  or cup
- **Lip retraction**: pulling back the lips in a very tight
  smile-like pattern at the approach of a stimulus toward the face
- **Nasal regurgitation**: movement of oral contents up
  into the nose and lower sinus during swallowing
- **Sensory defensiveness**: strong adverse reaction to
  touch, light, or sound

ASSESSMENT OF FEEDING PROBLEMS

To assess potential feeding problems, observe the caregiver feeding the child in a typical setting such as home
or school. Some children have more feeding and eating
problems in public than when they are at home. Observe
family members as they feed the child to determine if cues
or interactions are creating a problem. Support the less-
successful feeder so that a more positive feeding relation-
ship can be established. Also, consult with a speech and
language pathologist or occupational therapist. When the

RD observes a feeding session, many factors should be included in the observation and the accompanying interview to provide a complete assessment (see Box 3.6) (2).

Box 3.6   Nutrition Assessment of Feeding Problems

Observation
- Positioning
- Length of time of feeding
- Amount of food consumed
- Amount of liquid offered and consumed
- Appetite and signs of hunger or fullness
- Rate of eating and drinking
- How food is refused
- Feeding utensils used
- Interaction between the child and feeder

Interview Topics
- Types of food eaten
- Texture and consistency of foods
- Number of feedings per day
- Food allergies/intolerances
- Use of supplements, herbal preparations, and alternative therapies
- Sources of food and formulas, such as WIC, school, and other programs
- Medications taken
- Sources of family stress or concern, such as child care

Additional Considerations (2)
- Is the child independent for feeding or dependent on others?
- Does the child eat entirely by mouth or are supplemental tube feedings necessary?
- Does the feeding problem change from beginning to middle to end of the meal?
- Does the feeding problem vary with time of day or who is administering the meal?
- Does the feeding problem vary with social inclusion/who is eating with the child? For example another parent, sibling, friend, etc.

(continued)

Box 3.6   Nutrition Assessment of Feeding Problems (continued)

- Are there any signs of breathing difficulty during feeding?
- Does the child have emesis? If yes, when and how much?
- Does the child get irritable, sleepy, or lethargic during mealtime?

Abbreviation: WIC, Special Supplemental Nutrition Program for Women, Infants and Children.

If feeding concerns become apparent during the feeding observation and interview, the RD should determine whether the child would be an appropriate candidate for feeding therapy based on the "red flags" listed in Box 3.7.

Box 3.7   Red Flags: Is This Child a Candidate for Referral to a Feeding Specialist?

If any of the following are true for a patient, he or she should be referred to a feeding specialist:
- Ongoing poor weight gain or weight loss
- Ongoing choking, gagging, or coughing during meals
- Ongoing problems with vomiting
- More than one incident of nasal reflux
- History of a traumatic choking incident
- History of eating and breathing coordination problems, with ongoing respiratory issues
- Inability to transition to baby food purees by 10 months of age
- Inability to accept any table food solids by 12 months of age
- Inability to transition from breast/bottle to a cup by 16 months of age
- Has not weaned off baby foods by 16 months of age
- Aversion or avoidance of all foods in specific texture or food group
- Food range of less than 20 foods, especially if foods are being dropped over time with no new foods replacing those lost
- An infant who cries and/or arches at most meals

(continued)

Box 3.7   Red Flags: Is This Child a Candidate for Referral to a Feeding Specialist? (continued)

- Family is fighting about food and feeding (ie, meals are battles)
- Parent repeatedly reports that the child is difficult for everyone to feed
- Parental history of an eating disorder, with a child not meeting weight goals
- The child's social therapeutics or educational activities are limited (eg, the child who cannot attend a full day of school because he won't eat at school)

Source: Adapted with permission from Kay Toomey, PhD.

Feeding problems are often associated with a variety diagnoses and conditions; the most common are listed in Table 3.2 (4,8,9). The RD's ability to recognize behaviors and possible nutritional consequences is imperative when monitoring the nutrition status of patient(s) having said diagnoses.

Table 3.2   Common Diagnoses and Conditions Associated with Feeding Problems

Diagnosis	Behavior	Possible Nutritional Consequences
Autism	Rigid food acceptance; picky eating	Nutrient deficiency
Cerebral palsy	Swallowing difficulties; limited hunger cues; underfeeding	Failure to thrive
Down syndrome	Difficulty coordinating sucking, swallowing, and breathing during infancy; overfeeding/overeating in older children	Failure to thrive; overweight or obesity

(continued)

Table 3.2   Common Diagnoses and Conditions Associated with Feeding Problems (continued)

Diagnosis	Behavior	Possible Nutritional Consequences
Drug-exposed infants	Non-nutritive need to suck; overfeeding	Excessive weight gain
Fetal alcohol syndrome	Distorted hunger perception; undereating	Underweight
Prader-Willi syndrome	Weak oral skills, poor suck, hypotonia during infancy; distorted sense of hunger/satiety; overeating in older children	Suboptimal weight gain/growth; excessive weight gain or obesity
Premature or very low birth weight infant	Subtle and delayed hunger cues, difficult for parent to recognize	Sleepy or irritable infant with slow weight gain
Spina bifida	Overfeeding; overeating with limited activity; picky eating; difficulty swallowing in some cases	Overweight or obesity; nutrient deficiencies

Data are from references 4, 8, and 9.

PREMATURITY: FEEDING SKILL DEVELOPMENT AND BEHAVIOR

Infants who are healthy but premature and low-birth-weight have a range of feeding problems that are less likely to be seen in full-term infants. Accurate assessment, using corrected age, is useful in establishing nutritional and feeding goals and anticipating potential difficulties. Nutrient requirements of premature infants are generally higher than those of full-term infants because of limited body stores, metabolic and physiological immaturity, and increased growth rates (10). See Table 3.3 for developmental maturity and nutritional implications for premature infants (4,10).

Table 3.3   Developmental Maturity and Nutritional Implications for Premature Infants

Common Presentations in Prematurity	Resultant Problems
Immature suck-swallow-breathe coordination emerges between 33 and 36 weeks gestational age	Impaired nippling ability; increased risk of aspiration; decreased feeding efficiency; fatigue
Diminished or absent gag and cough reflex	Increased risk of aspiration
Decreased muscle tone	Inability to maintain optimal feeding position; decline in swallow function
Neurological and behavioral immaturity	Subtle cues of hunger, satiety, and distress; more time spent sleeping; less time alert for feedings; disorganized feeding skills
Immature peristaltic and gastrointestinal motility patterns	Delayed gastric emptying; increased transit time; constipation
Decreased or absent sucking pads	Decreased sucking strength and stamina
Reduced gastric volume	Volume limitations
Alterations in renal and cardiac function	Fluid and electrolyte imbalance; alteration in protein tolerance

Data are from references 4 and 10.

Effects of extended hospitalization on premature infants can include the following:

• Infant–caregiver bonding time could be limited due to the infant's medical fragility.

- Opportunities for parents to feed infants may be limited for a variety of reasons; NICU babies are often also fed by multiple nurses and sometimes even volunteers.
- Parents may be anxious about weight gain as this is often final criteria for hospital discharge.
- Some infants experience set-backs in feeding and growth.
- Nipple feeding may increase energy expenditure in some infants.
- Some premature infants have had negative oral experiences or limited mouth play, making them extra-sensitive to changes in their mouths (4).

Ways to promote feeding for premature infants are outlined in Table 3.4 (1,11–14).

Table 3.4   Ways to Promote Feeding for Premature Infants

What to Do	What to Expect
Offer breastmilk, fortified breastmilk, or nutritionally appropriate formula	Appropriate weight gain and growth
Offer small, frequent meals	Increased daily intake as some infants are volume sensitive
Create a calm feeding environment	A quiet room and low light decrease risk for potential distractions while feeding
Help prepare infant for feeding	Swaddling and thumb sucking soothes the infant
Establish a position to improve suck	Chin tucked slightly, head supported, one or both arms forward, straight trunk and bent hips help improve intake

(continued)

Table 3.4   Ways to Promote Feeding for Premature Infants
(continued)

What to Do	What to Expect
Support jaw	Improves infant's ability to latch on to breast or nipple of the bottle
Try special feeding equipment	Soft nipple or angle-necked bottle decreases effort required for feeding

Source: Data are from references 1 and 11–14.

GASTROESOPHAGEAL REFLUX DISEASE: FEEDING DEVELOPMENT AND BEHAVIOR

In addition to the diagnoses listed in Table 3.2, gastro-esophageal reflux disease (GERD), fluid and bowel problems, and neuromuscular disorders may also interfere with feeding development and behavior. GERD is a condition in which the contents of the stomach seep back into the esophagus and/or throat (4). It occurs when the sphincter between the stomach and esophagus is not mature or does not function properly.

When stomach contents seep into the throat and enter the child's airway, this can cause aspiration, which leads to spitting, vomiting, or retching. Some indications of GERD include the following:

- Refusal to eat
- Stops eating after only a small amount of food is taken
- Cries and/or becomes irritable during feeding
- Use of other behavior to communicate their distress

Infants typically often outgrow GERD by 12 to 18 months of age. However, children with neurological impairments are often diagnosed after infancy, when reflux may continue and be more severe (1). The condition can vary over time from dormancy to active irritation in some children. The effectiveness of nonsurgical treatments such as positioning and thickened feedings has been disputed (15). Secondhand smoke can alter lower esophageal sphincter pressure and promote reflux (16). Table 3.5 outlines nutrition assessment and intervention considerations related to GERD (1,17).

Table 3.5   Nutrition Assessment and Interventions Related to Gastroesophageal Reflux Disease

Assessment	Possible Interventions
History of frequent spitting up, choking, coughing, or difficulties with breathing during and after meals	Upright positioning; elevated sleeping position
Food refusal	Change mealtime volume and timing (smaller, more frequent feedings)
History of repeated upper respiratory infections and pneumonia	Thicken liquids and foods
Positive finding on upper gastrointestinal (UGI) studies, pH probe or in response to medication	Prescription medications; surgical correction such as fundoplication

Source: Data are from references 1 and 17.

FLUID AND BOWEL PROBLEMS: FEEDING DEVELOPMENT AND BEHAVIOR

Children with special health care needs have the same problems with fluid and bowel management as other children, but encounter these problems more often. Some children find drinking less fatiguing than consuming solid foods, often resulting in decreased nutrient intake provided by solids. Other children having difficulty consuming liquids are at risk for dehydration and constipation. Some chronic conditions are sensitive to fluid balance and can worsen with low fluid intakes. For some children with feeding difficulties, fluid intake is low because liquids are more difficult to handle in the mouth and can cause choking. High fluid needs may relate to drooling or oral losses while eating, but liquids should not replace more nutritionally dense foods unless these are planned supplements (18).

NEUROMUSCULAR PROBLEMS: FEEDING DEVELOPMENT AND BEHAVIOR

Children with neuromuscular problems may need a quiet environment with few distracting elements. These children have less control of their muscles when they are in highly stimulating environments. This can increase the work associated with eating. Muscle relaxants for spasticity may affect swallowing function in addition to targeted muscles.

SWALLOWING PROBLEMS

Swallowing problems are common among children with special health care needs and must be carefully assessed so as to identify the child's degree of risk for aspiration. RDs are encouraged to approach their medical team when swallowing problems appear to be present following feeding observations. A referral for an evaluation by a speech and language pathologist (SLP) may be appropriate.

Swallowing dysfunction can lead to aspiration, decreased food intake and impact on overall health. A swallow study may be recommended to determine risk for aspiration and need for appropriate food texture. Some children better organize swallowing of thickened liquids. Some children's swallowing abilities change over time particularly with correction of failure to thrive and improved head positioning. Repeat swallow studies are recommended if parents believe there have been changes. Tables 3.6 and 3.7 explain the anatomy of swallowing and the phases of swallowing (7).

Table 3.6   The Anatomy of Swallowing

Anatomical Feature	Role in Swallowing
Oral cavity—upper jaw (maxilla), lower jaw (mandible), upper/ lower lips, cheeks, tongue, teeth, hard/soft palates, uvula, anterior/ posterior facial arches	Sucking and suckling; biting; chewing
Pharynx—pharyngeal constrictors	Swallowing; functions as a valve at the top of the esophagus
Larynx	Prevents food from entering the airway
Esophagus (23–25 cm long)	Propels food boluses by peristaltic movements
Lower esophageal sphincter	Prevents regurgitation of stomach contents back into the esophagus

Source: Data are from reference 7.

Table 3.7   The Phases of Swallowing

Phase	Description
Oral	Food or liquid is organized into a bolus and moved from the front to the back of the mouth. Bolus is held and released to the pharynx as the swallow is triggered.

(continued)

Table 3.7   The Phases of Swallowing (continued)

Phase	Description
Pharyngeal	The nasal, laryngeal, and oral openings close to prevent fluid leakage. Bolus is channeled into the esophagus.
Esophageal	Peristaltic contractions move the fluid or bolus toward the stomach.

Source: Data are from reference 7.

Evaluation of Swallowing

The appropriate examination technique depends on which anatomic areas and functional processes need to be assessed. The following are commonly used assessment methods (2,19):

- **Videofluoroscopic swallow study (VFSS)**: a primary technique for detailed dynamic imaging of oral, pharyngeal, and upper esophageal phases of swallowing, VFSS issued primarily for diagnostic purposes. This is also known as *upper modified barium swallow*.
- **Fiberoptic endoscopic examination of swallowing (FEES)**: often performed by otolaryngologist and speech-language pathologist (SLP), FEES can include sensory testing (FEESST). FEES helps clarify oral feeding status, particularly in children with developmental disabilities and is used to assess laryngeal function and airway protection, as well as possible anatomic factors, and aspiration risk of even minute amounts of material. FEES is a more conservative approach than VFSS as barium is not used when the patient is at increased risk of aspiration. The procedure requires that a flexible endoscope be

passed transnasally into the oropharynx where the examiner can clearly view anatomic structures and laryngeal function.

- **Ultrasound**: Ultrasound is most helpful in describing oral preparatory and oral phases of swallowing, especially in young infants.
- **Pharyngeal manometry**: The best method for evaluating pharyngeal and esophageal motor function, this procedure requires insertion of a catheter with a series of intraluminal transducers.

Box 3.8 identifies nutrition assessment findings and possible interventions for swallowing dysfunction (1,8,21).

Box 3.8   Nutrition Assessment and Interventions for Swallowing Dysfunction

---

Nutrition Assessment
- History of frequent spitting up, choking, coughing, or difficulties with breathing during and after meals
- History of repeated upper respiratory infections and pneumonia
- Noisy or wet sounding upper airway sounds
- Drooling or pooling of saliva
- More than one swallow needed to clear a bolus

Possible Interventions
- Evaluate the feeding pace and positions that enhance safe swallowing.
- Refer child to a speech, occupational therapist, or feeding team for specific feeding techniques.
- Consider swallow study to determine if child is at risk for aspiration.
- If aspiration is documented, refer for non-oral feeding interventions or instruct on appropriate thickening for safety.

Source: Data are from references 1, 8, 20, and 21.

Use of Thickeners

If the child is diagnosed with dysphagia, thickening agents will likely be added to food and/or liquid with hopes of slowing the bolus when swallowed and preventing aspiration (see Tables 3.8 and 3.9) (21). The speech-language pathologist (SLP) will determine the appropriate thickness based on the patient's degree of dysphagia. Thickness of liquids can range from nectar to honey to pudding thick. It is also important to keep in mind that the caloric intake from thickeners can be significant and contribute to excessive weight gain.

Table 3.8   Widely Available Food Thickeners

Food	*Calories/Tbsp*	*Used with Liquids*	*Used with Foods*
Pureed or blenderized fruits and vegetables	5–11	X	
Infant cereal	15	X	X
Yogurt	8–15	X	
Soft tofu	10	X	
Potato flakes	11		X
Bread crumbs	22		X

Source: Data are from reference 23.

Table 3.9   Commercial Thickening Agents to Be Used with
Liquids and Foods

Product	Calories
Powders	
Thick-It	15/Tbsp
Thick-it II	20/Tbsp
Thick and Easy	15/Tbsp
Thicken Up	15/Tbsp
Nutrathik (includes 19 vitamins and minerals)	20/Tbsp
Gels	
Simply Thick (nectar), 15-g packet	0/packet
Simply Thick (honey), 30-g packet	0/packet
Hydra-Aid (nectar), 12-g packet	0/packet
Hydra-Aid (honey), 26-g packet	5/packet

Source: Data are from reference 23.

Some thickeners bind part of the fluid consumed, decreasing bioavailability. Water intake must be assessed in children with special health care needs. Poor hydration can lead to constipation, concentration of urine, and dehydration.

Keep in mind that fluid problems can progress to medical emergencies in vulnerable children. Immediate referral back to the child's pediatrician, specialty health care team, or emergency service is appropriate for some children. Children who should be referred include those with a history of dehydration or fluid overload for pulmonary or cardiac problems requiring prescribed medications such as furosemide (Lasix). Oral rehydration therapy

(ORT) or intravenous fluids may be medically necessary if early signs of dehydration are not identified (18).

EFFECTS OF MEDICATIONS ON FEEDING AND EATING

Many children with special health care needs take multiple medications. These may present challenges to feeding, eating, and nutritional status. It is important to review medication lists regularly as nutrition concerns may appear following the introduction of a new medication. Medications can have the following effects on feeding and eating (4,22):

- Depress or increase appetite
- Distort taste
- Reduce alertness
- Alter the swallow reflex
- Cause nausea
- Produce dryness of the oral mucosa
- Irritate the gastrointestinal tract
- Result in malabsorption of nutrients
- Cause constipation

GUIDELINES FOR SUCCESSFUL FEEDING AND EATING

Feeding is successful when the caregiver attends to the child's rhythm and signals of hunger and satiety, works to calm him/her, and develops mechanics of feeding that are effective with the child's particular emotional makeup, skill, and limitations. Many caregivers perceive total oral intake as a marker of success. Some children, however, require tube feedings to better meet nutrition and hydration needs without placing undue risk on the respiratory system and/or the energy levels required for feeding orally (2). A sense of failure, following the placement of a feeding tube, is often reported by caregivers who hope their child could be an oral feeder. Thus, it is important for caregivers to understand that feeding therapy requires time just like any other behavior change. Some families work on feeding for a while and then stop. Leave the door open to try therapy again, as the family's coping abilities permit. Each family has its own "comfort foods" that are associated with fun and caring. Try to incorporate these foods into feeding interventions to make feeding and eating a positive experience for the family.

The following three components should be in place to support oral nutrition (5):

- **Physical**: getting the food to your mouth, moving it around in your mouth and swallowing it
- **Sensory**: managing the smell, taste, feel, sight, and sound of food
- **Emotional**: managing how you feel about eating

In addition, body position should be monitored to support feeding success. See Box 3.9 for guidelines for optimal feeding position (14,24).

Box 3.9   Guidelines for Optimal Feeding Position

- Head is midline.
- Head and neck are in neutral position.
- Knees are bent.
- Feet are supported.
- Sitting balance is stable and supported if necessary.
- Sitting in a semi-upright position (infants).

Source: Data are from references 14 and 24.

Learning the Stages of Eating

Eating is a learned behavior requiring a series of fundamental steps that must be completed sequentially in order for eating to be successful. Oftentimes parents are discouraged when their child regresses to a previous step. It is important to support the parent and child as each step should be treated as a monumental accomplishment. The Sensory Stages of Eating (Box 3.10) are designed to promote the acceptance of new foods by slowly overcoming aversion to the presence, smell, texture and taste of foods (4). Common types of food refusal are outlined in Box 3.11 (9,25). These limitations in diet can result in deficiencies of key nutrients.

Box 3.10   Sensory Stages of Eating

Step 1: Accepts the Presence of Food
- Allows food to be present on plate/tray
- Can be in the same room as others with the food
- Can watch others eat the food
- Can sit at the table with the food in a serving bowl or on another's plate

Step 2: Accepts the Odor of Food
- Allows food to touch plate
- Allows food to be on table in serving bowl
- Can be present when food is cooking in the kitchen

Step 3: Explores the Properties of Food
- Touches food to tongue, lips, near nose
- Holds food in whole hand
- Touches food with fingers (throws onto the floor)
- Touches food with utensil

(continued)

Box 3.10 Sensory Stages of Eating (continued)

Step 4: Samples the Food
- Chews and swallows easily
- Chews, swallows, and follows with a drink immediately
- Bites off a small piece and starts to chew before spitting out
- Licks food

Step 5: Eats the Food
- Successfully consumes food in its entirety

Source: Adapted with permission from "Steps to Eating" by Kay Toomey, PhD, Denver, CO.

Box 3.11 Feeding Concerns and Possible Solutions

Refusal to Eat Meat
- Incorporate meat in spaghetti sauce, stews, casseroles, burritos, pizza.
- Offer legumes, eggs, cheese, tofu and boneless fish (canned tuna and salmon), cottage cheese, yogurt.
- Use wet-cook methods for preparing meats.

Refusal to Drink Milk
- Offer cheese, yogurt, cream soups, milk-based puddings.
- Use milk to cook hot cereals.
- Include cheese in cooking (sauces, pizza, macaroni and cheese).
- Allow child to pour milk from container and use a straw.
- Use powdered milk in cooking and baking (biscuits, muffins, pancakes, meat loaf, casseroles).
- Consider adding small amounts of flavored syrups.
- Offer beverages fortified with calcium and vitamin D as alternatives.

Excessive Intake of Milk
- Limit milk to one serving with meals; offer water for seconds.
- Offer milk at end of meal.
- Offer water if thirsty between meals.

(continued)

Box 3.11   Feeding Concerns and Possible Solutions (continued)

Refusal to Eat Fruits and Vegetables
- Prepare vegetables that are tender, but not overcooked.
- Steam vegetables (or offer raw if appropriate) and allow child to eat with fingers.
- Offer sauces/dips.
- Mix vegetable purees into soups/sauces, hamburgers, meat loaf, or meatballs.
- Add dried fruit to cereal or trail mixes (use with children >3 years of age to prevent choking risk).
- Prepare fruit in a variety of ways (fresh, cooked, juice, gelatin, salad).
- Add fruit purees into mixes (pancakes, waffles, and muffins).
- Mix fruit purees into yogurt, milkshakes, and pudding to add flavor.
- Bring child along to the store to select a new fruit or vegetable he/she would like to try.
- Have the child help prepare the food.
- Continue to offer a variety despite refusal.

Excessive Intake of Sweet Foods
- Limit availability of sweet foods in the home.
- Avoid using sweets as a bribe or reward at home, in therapy, and/or school.
- Incorporate into meals instead of snacks for better dental health.
- Decrease amount of sugar used in recipes by half.
- Consider working with daycare/school staff regarding provision of treats while away from home.

Source: Data are from references 9 and 25.

Scheduling Tips

Children with special needs often benefit from structured daily schedules. The likelihood that children may consume a meal may be increased by scheduling meal times when they are at their best. Suggestions for scheduling meals include the following:

- Regular structured times for meals, snacks, bed, and naps are necessary for most children.
- Most children will not eat if overly tired.
- Most children with congestion will eat less in the morning when congestion is worse.
- Children need snacks; five to six meals and snacks per day are common for young children.

Presentation of Food Tips

Presentation of foods can also be a critical component when feeding problems exist. Creativity and exploration of the child's taste preferences is often necessary. The following tips can be helpful:

- Offer small servings
- Offer foods that are separate rather than mixed
- Serve foods at mild temperatures
- Choose bright colors (attract interest)
- Choose bland flavors (for infants)
- Choose sharper, spicier flavors (for older children)

Guidelines for Child's Feeding Environment

The feeding environment is important to children and families. The following factors require consideration to support optimal feeding (14,24):

- Child is comfortable and feels safe.
- Feeder can focus attention on child.
- Noise level in the room is not distracting (eg, school cafeterias).
- Items that distract the child from eating (eg, television and toys) are minimized.
- Temperature of the room is comfortable.
- Lighting is adequate.

Feeding Tips for Caregivers

The following tips may help caregivers feel more comfortable and garner greater success in feeding their children:

- Face the child to make eye contact at his/her level.
- Try to keep the level of anxiety about eating low.
- Set a comfortable pace and length for the meal.
- Smile and praise the child for small successful steps.
- Identify positive attention-seeking behaviors and respond with attention; this behavior may not be related to hunger.
- Ignore negative, attention-seeking behaviors.
- Try to be consistent; avoid over- and under-reacting.
- Read nonverbal, as well as verbal, signs from the child.
- Do not use food as a reward; positive attention is a better reward.
- Seek support for feelings of anger, sadness, or frustration at mealtimes.

REFERRAL FOR FEEDING PROBLEMS: FEEDING TEAMS

Assessment of feeding problems is most effectively done with an interdisciplinary team approach. It is important to refer a child to a specialty interdisciplinary team for assistance when feeding and eating problems are beyond the usual level of difficulties.

A parent who is frustrated, angry, and feeling unsuccessful in caring for a child is likely to be considered noncompliant, but may simply need additional support. Frustration due to lack of progress in feeding and eating will delay more effective interventions that could be identified by a feeding team. To distinguish between physical, behavioral, and interaction problems an interdisciplinary team approach is often helpful (26). The team may be comprised of the following members:

- Registered dietitian (RD)
- Speech-language pathologist (SLP)
- Occupational therapist (OT)
- Physical therapist (PT)
- Registered nurse (RN)
- Social worker
- Pediatric gastroenterologist
- Developmental pediatrician
- Radiologist
- Psychologist or behavioral specialist

A list of services provided by feeding teams is found in Box 3.12 (7,26,27).

Box 3.12 Services Provided by Feeding Teams

- Observe eating or feeding to assess and make recommendations for improving oral feeding.
- Order appropriate tests such as the modified barium swallow to confirm that oral feeding is safe.
- Assess nutritional status and growth and provide appropriate interventions.
- Assess for behavior-based feeding difficulties and provide therapy.
- Recommend appropriate oral-feeding methods to stimulate oral-skill development.
- Monitor intervention therapies at school or programs to maximize skills.
- Follow-up with the child over time to assess growth and progress in developing feeding skills.

Source: Data are from references 7, 26, and 27.

Ways to Access a Feeding Team

Feeding teams can be accessed in the following ways (7,26,27):

- Through local early intervention program (birth to 3 years of age) or special education department of the school system
- Through a pediatric hospital or facility with pediatric specialties
- By contacting a local health department or other community programs with services for high-risk infants and children with special health care needs

Feeding Team Interventions

Feeding team interventions may include a variety of techniques discussed in this chapter, including the following (7,27):

- Ensuring the proper positioning of the child during feeding, with home and school devices prescribed by appropriate physicians and related providers
- Instruction in special feeding techniques and use of utensils such as scoop plates or built-up spoons for self-feeding
- Recommendations of specific food textures and consistencies for stimulation oral-motor sensations and chewing
- Establishment of energy goals plus meal and snack schedules for behavior and attention problems that interfere with eating
- Adjusting the nutrient density and consistency of food choices to maximize oral-motor skills and decrease fatigue

- Oral-motor therapy techniques outside of meal times for some problems, such as proprioceptive integration
- Referral for proprioceptive or neurophysiologic approaches as appropriate
- Therapy for specific oral-motor problems, such as muscle relaxation techniques for the upper lip
- Identifying and supporting positive parent–child feeding interactions
- Parenting education or family counseling, as appropriate
- Additional diagnostic tests and medical interventions such as medications to reduce salivary gland secretions

SUMMARY

Children with special health care needs are at increased risk of encountering feeding difficulties. To promote successful growth, families should be observant of the child's eating patterns. When feedings become stressful as a result of battling with the child to consume a meal, professional assistance should be sought to assess the situation. Feeding difficulties do not have to consume the daily life of the child and or family members, and can be managed with the support of interdisciplinary team members.

REFERENCES

1. Morris SE. *Pre-feeding Skills: A Comprehensive Resource for Feeding Development*. Tucson, AZ: Therapy Skill Builders; 1997.
2. Arvedson JC, Rudolph CD. Feeding and swallowing issues relevant to pediatric nutrition support. In: Baker SS, Baker RD,

Davis AM. *Pediatric Nutrition Support.* Sudbury, MA: Jones and Bartlett Publishers; 2007:149–58.

3. Akers S, Groh-Wargo S. Normal nutrition during infancy. In: Samour PQ, King K. *Handbook of Pediatric Nutrition.* 3rd ed. Sudbury, MA: Jones and Bartlett Publishers; 2005:75–106.

4. Nardella M, Campo L, Ogata B, eds. *Nutrition Interventions for Children with Special Health Care Needs.* Olympia, WA: Washington State Department of Health; 2002.

5. Medlen JE. *The Down Syndrome Nutrition Handbook: A Guide to Promoting Healthy Lifestyles.* Bethesda, MD: Woodbine House; 2002.

6. Barnard K. *NCAST Feeding Scale.* Seattle, WA: NCAST Publications, University of Washington School of Nursing; 1994.

7. Cloud H, Ekvall SW, Hicks L. Feeding problems of the child with special health care needs. In: Ekvall SW, Ekvall VK. *Pediatric Nutrition in Chronic Disease and Developmental Disorders: Prevention, Assessment, and Treatment.* 2nd ed. New York, NY: Oxford University Press: 2005:172–181.

8. Pipes PL, Glass R. Nutrition and special health care needs. In: Trahms CM, Pipes PL, eds. *Nutrition in Infancy and Childhood.* 6th ed. Columbus, OH: WCN/McGraw-Hill; 1997: 377–405.

9. Owens A, Cloud HP. Special topics in toddler and preschool nutrition: vitamins and minerals in childhood and children with disabilities. In: Edelstein S, Sharlin J. *Life Cycle Nutrition: An Evidence-based Approach.* Sudbury, MA: Jones and Bartlett Publishers; 2009:204–220.

10. Anderson DM. Nutrition for premature infants. In: Samour PQ and King K. *Handbook of Pediatric Nutrition.* 3rd ed. Sudbury, MA: Jones and Bartlett Publishers; 2005:53–73.

11 Dunn M, Delaney T. *Feeding and Nutrition for the Child with Special Health Needs.* Tucson, AZ: Therapy Skill Builders; 1994.

12. Carlson S, Armentrout C. *Neonatal Nutrition Handbook.* Iowa City, IA: University of Iowa Hospitals and Clinics Dietary Department; 1994.

13. *Feeding Management of a Child with a Handicap: A Guide for Professionals.* Knoxville, TN: University of Tennessee; 1990.

14. Howard RB, Winter HS. *Nutrition and Feeding Infants and Toddlers*. Boston, MA: Little Brown; 1994.

15. Carroll A, Garrison M, Christakis D. A systematic review of nonpharmacological and nonsurgical therapies for gastroesophageal reflux in infants. *Arch Pediatr Adolesc Med*. 2002; 152:109–113.

16. Locke GR 3rd, Talley NJ, Fett SL, et al. Risk factors associated with symptoms of gastroesophageal reflux. *Am J Med*. 1999;106:642–649.

17. Zerzan J, Glass R. Evaluating the young child who presents with growth concerns and feeding difficulties. *Nutr Focus*. 1996;11(2):1–8.

18. Nardella MT, Owens-Kuehner A. Feeding and eating. In: Lucas B. *Children with Special Health Care Needs: Nutrition Care Handbook*. Chicago, IL: American Dietetic Association; 2004:59–85.

19. Kleinman RE. *Pediatric Nutrition Handbook*. 5th ed. Elk Grove, IL: American Academy of Pediatrics; 2004.

20. Lowman DK, Murphy SM, Snell ME. *The Educator's Guide to Feeding Children with Disabilities*. Baltimore, MD: Paul H Brookes Publishing; 1998.

21. Department of Nutrition and Food Service. *Pediatric Nutrition Handbook*. 3rd ed. Boston, MA: Children's Hospital; 1993.

22. Pronsky ZM, Powers DE. *Powers and Moore's Food Medication Interactions*. 11th ed. Birchrunville, PA: Food-Medication Interactions; 2000.

23. Feucht S. Thickening foods for children. *Nutr Focus*. 2003; 18(5):1–6.

24. Taylor S, Wheeler LC, Taylor JR. Nutrition: an issue of concern for children with disabilities. *Nurs Pract*. 1996;21(10):17-18,20.

25. Lucas B, Ogata B. Normal nutrition from infancy through adolescence. In: Samour PQ, King K. *Handbook of Pediatric Nutrition*. 3rd ed. Sudbury, MA: Jones and Bartlett; 2005:107–130.

26. Wodarski LA. An interdisciplinary nutrition assessment and intervention protocol for children with disabilities. *J Am Diet Assoc*. 1990;90:1563–1568.

27. Hendricks K, Walker W. *Manual of Pediatric Nutrition*. 3rd ed. Philadelphia, PA: BC Decker; 2000.

Chapter 4

Non-Oral Enteral Feeding

Marion Taylor Baer, PhD, RD,
Cary B. Kreutzer, MPH, RD,
L. Hope Wills, MA, RD, CSP, CLS, and
Mildred K. Leatham, MPH, RD, CHES

Enteral nutrition (EN) is recommended when a child has a functional gastrointestinal (GI) tract but is either unable to consume adequate nutrients by mouth or at risk for aspiration when swallowing (1,2). EN can be used for both short-term rehabilitation and long-term nutrition management. Non-oral or EN provides nutrition using the GI tract using a tube, catheter, or stoma to deliver nutrients (3). Some children benefit from supplementary EN when they are unable to meet all their nutrient needs by mouth (4). Benefits of EN include improved growth and nutritional status to ensure that nutrient needs are met; improved hydration and bowel function; and the ability to provide consistent medication administration.

Non-oral feeding systems have various devices that are used for infusion. Types of EN are named according to the feeding route used and the point at which nutrients are delivered, including gastrostomy, or G-tube, for direct feedings into the stomach; jejunostomy, or J-tube, for feedings delivered into the jejunum; and transpyloric for feedings delivered into the duodenum. A gastrojejunostomy or GJ-tube is inserted into the wall of the stomach with two ports. One port is inserted into the stomach for fluids, medications, and venting. The other is inserted into the jejunum for continuous feeding for patients who require long-term EN and have delayed gastric emptying, GE reflux, or risk for aspiration (2). Tube feedings can be administered as bolus feeding, continuous drip or a combination of the two along with oral intake.

Individualized nutrient needs, delivery route, and formula type are defined by the registered dietitian (RD) working in partnership with the health care team or, in the optimal situation, a specialized feeding team. The individualized EN plan should take into account the diagnosis, GI function, nutrient requirements, medications, key laboratory test results, and family social factors (5).

Note: This chapter does *not* cover parenteral nutrition support, which is indicated when a child does not have a functioning GI tract (eg, total parenteral nutrition) or when specialized modular components are administered via the bloodstream.

FAMILY CONCERNS

Feeding a child is an expression of love and nurturing. Being unable to feed a child by mouth can undermine feelings of competence in parents (6,7). Many parents resist initial discussions of non-oral feeding. Providing the family with the rationale to support non-oral feeding, including potential risks and benefits, while acknowledging the difficult decision the family must make, will support the emotional coping required (7). Some families may request EN access to infuse fluids or medications, or to provide nutrition when their child is sick and not able to eat.

The timing of the well-thought out decision to begin EN placement needs to be made as early as possible. Rushing the parents into a decision may result in poor cooperation and inadequate use of the feeding support system. Conversely, if a child is undernourished due to inadequate intake, delaying the decision too long increases the risk for complications related to malnutrition. Family support groups or talking with another parent of a child receiving EN may help reassure parents. Web sites that may be helpful to both the health care professionals and to families are listed in Box 4.1.

Box 4.1   Useful Web-based Resources

Resources for Health Care Professionals
- Academy of Nutrition and Dietetics Pediatric Nutrition Practice Group: www.pnpg.org
- American Society for Parenteral and Enteral Nutrition (ASPEN): www.nutritioncare.org
- Oley Foundation: www.oley.org
- Pediatric/Adolescent Gastroesophageal Reflux Association (PAGER): www.reflux.org
- University of Washington. Gaining and Growing: Assuring Nutritional Care of Preterm Infants. http://depts.washington.edu/growing

Resources for Parents and Caregivers
- Children with Disabilities: www.childrensdisabilities.info/feeding/groups-feeding-children.html
- Kids Health (search for gastrostomy, enteral): www.kidshealth.org
- Our Kids: www.our-kids.org

NON-ORAL FEEDING DEVICES AND SPECIALTY FEEDING TEAMS

Many conditions, such as undernutrition, aspiration, and risks related to coordination of breathing and eating, result in recommendations for non-oral feeding (7–9).

Diagnoses that require prolonged hospitalizations, are degenerative, or have a neurological component, routinely necessitate EN. In some disorders, such as cystic fibrosis or cerebral palsy, the need for EN may increase as functional skills decrease or risk for aspiration increases. In other instances, for example, craniofacial malformations, the need for EN is indicated prior to surgical repair and may not be needed following surgery. The need for long-term or lifetime EN may be present in children with inborn errors of metabolism or anatomic abnormalities in the airway, face, upper intestinal tract, or neuromuscular disorders (10).

There are a number of presenting signs and symptoms that indicate a need for enteral nutrition. Box 4.2 lists common clinical signs and reported family concerns that are indicators for EN (3,5,11).

Box 4.2   Signs and Symptoms Requiring Consideration of Non-oral Feeding

Clinical Observation
- Inability to consume at least 80% of estimated energy needs or 90% of fluid needs by mouth, over an extended period of time
- Fatigue
- Indicators of malnutrition as defined through laboratory indices, especially long-term indicators
- Anthropometric measurements and growth history
- Repeated unexplained upper-airway infections or pneumonia
- Patient "failing" one or more modified barium swallow studies
- History of gastroesophageal reflux, failed medical treatment
- History of weight loss or deceleration in weight gain, associated with illness or surgery that does not correct with oral feeding

(continued)

**Box 4.2   Signs and Symptoms Requiring Consideration of
Non-oral Feeding** (continued)

Family Concerns
- Prolonged feeding time (> 4 h/d)
- Food refusal or a poor appetite for favorite foods
- Frequent meal interruptions due to distraction, discomfort (loud crying, coughing)
- Hearing a "wet cough" or congestion after feeding or other signs of aspiration
- Change of skin color, retching, vomiting, or other signs of distress with feeding or eating

Source: Data are from references 3, 5, and 11.

There are multiple methods to gain enteral access for feeding, including surgical (laparotomy, laparoscopy), gastroenterological (endoscopy), and radiological (fluoroscopy) (3). Gastrostomy tube insertion is the most commonly used method for long-term enteral access and is inserted laparoscopically, often in combination with a Nissen fundoplication if reflux is a risk factor for the infant/child. The large diameter of the tube allows other functions including gastric pH monitoring, provision of viscous feedings, and medication delivery. A *percutaneous endoscopic gastrostomy* (PEG) is placed endoscopically under general anesthesia, requiring less than an hour for placement. The patient is sedated, and an endoscope is passed through the mouth and esophagus into the stomach, for placement of the external PEG entry site (3,10). Box 4.3 provides an outline of different feeding sites and their indications for use (1–3,12). Figure 4.1 is a decision tree model to help determine when non-oral feeding is indicated and the appropriate route for feeding.

Box 4.3   Non-oral Feeding Sites and Rationale for Use

Nasogastric or Orogastric
- Nutrients are delivered through a tube inserted via the nose or mouth into the stomach.
- Indicated for short term use (<4 weeks) in children who fail to demonstrate growth in the presence of adequate nutrition, following surgery or traumatic injury. Orogastric tubes are used only in critical-care settings combined with mechanical ventilation.
- Risks include dislodging (eg, child pulling out) and increased secretions.
- Simplest and least expensive.

Gastrostomy
- Nutrients are delivered directly into the stomach through a PEG or G-tube.
- Indicated for children who can't meet their nutritional needs by oral feeding alone due to chronic illness or feeding dysfunction.
- Intended for long-term use (> 4 weeks).

Duodenal
- Nutrients are delivered into the duodenum; tube is inserted past the pyloric sphincter.
- Indicated for children with moderate to severe reflux with vomiting or delayed gastric emptying, to reduce movement of the tube and avoid erosion of the esophagus.

Jejunostomy
- Nutrients are delivered into the jejunum by a tube passed through the stomach into the jejunum (GJ) or by a tube placed surgically directly into the jejunum (J-tube).
- Indicated for children with severe reflux, delayed gastric emptying, or poor tolerance of nutrients delivered into the stomach.

Source: Data are from references 1–3, and 12.

Figure 4.1   Enteral access decision tree. Abbreviations: PEG, percutaneous endoscopic gastrostomy; PEG/J, PEG with jejunal extension. Reprinted with permission from *ADA Pocket Guide to Enteral Nutrition* (3).

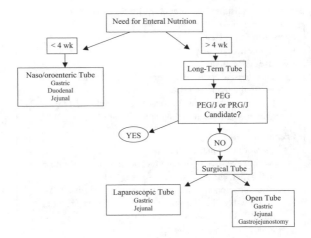

A specialty feeding team should ideally be involved in decision making for non-oral feeding, assessing patient needs for EN, developing a feeding plan, and defining nutrient needs. Box 4.4 provides examples of medical conditions that often warrant EN (1,3,5,7,12–14), and Box 4.5 identifies the team members who may be involved in EN. These specialists provide interdisciplinary, coordinated, and comprehensive care. Families may be unable to travel to see the specialty feeding team, as they are usually located in major pediatric centers or university hospitals. It is important to recognize the importance of a team approach, which is critical to ensuring optimal treatment for non-oral feeding. Community dietitians may help coordinate care for families living a distance from the specialty team. Members of the specialty feeding team each have a role in supporting the child and his or her family.

Box 4.4   Conditions That May Require Non-oral Feeding

Neuromuscular Disorders
- Examples: Cerebral palsy, muscular dystrophy
- Causes of inadequate oral intake:
    ◦ Poor muscle coordination of oral structures and swallowing so that there is a risk of aspiration
    ◦ Muscle weakness in oral structures, which interfere with chewing and increase fatigue while eating

Prematurity
- Causes of inadequate oral intake:
    ◦ Negative associations with the mouth that have resulted in oral hypersensitivity that causes gagging
    ◦ Underdeveloped or premature oral-motor skills (suck-swallow-breathe) causing inadequate intake (typical in infant < 32–34 weeks' gestational age)
    ◦ Risk for aspiration or reflux

Neurodevelopmental Disorders
- Example: Autism
- Causes of inadequate oral intake:
    ◦ Food texture avoidance
    ◦ Sensitivity to flavors, temperature, and appearance
    ◦ Poor motor planning

Genetic Disorders
- Examples: Down syndrome, metabolic disorders, mitochondrial disorders
- Causes of inadequate oral intake:
    ◦ Delayed acquisition of feeding skills due to developmental delay
    ◦ Central hypotonia that results in oral motor weakness
    ◦ Necessary diet and nutrient modifications required for management of specific disorders

(continued)

Box 4.4   Conditions That May Require Non-oral Feeding
(continued)

Genetic Disorders (continued)
- ○ Congenital malformations (eg, cleft lip/palate, trachea-esophageal fistula)
- ○ Anatomical malformation that impairs child's ability to meet nutritional requirements

Source: Data are from references 1, 3, 5, 7, and 12–14.

Box 4.5   Roles and Responsibilities of Specialty Team Members

- **Parent**: Provide information and direction to the team on the appropriate means to provide services for their child. This will be influenced by family preference and resources.
- **Primary physician**: Supervises the assessment process, making referrals to the appropriate disciplines to ensure a thorough evaluation, monitoring the outcomes of the evaluations and sharing findings with other team members (including the family).
- **Specialty medical** (eg, gastroenterology, radiology, pulmonology): Evaluate structure and function of the GI system; based on the evaluation, make recommendations for the type of feeding tube to place and assess pulmonary function prior to placement of the feeding tube.
- **Occupational therapist/speech language pathologist**: Evaluate oral feeding for coordination, effort, and safety. Participate and/or conduct a swallow study to determine patient swallowing abilities and safety. Provide ongoing support when feeding therapy is indicated.
- **Psychology and child development specialist**: Assist and support the family in normalizing the feeding experience.
- **Registered dietitian**: Define nutrition requirements and monitor intake to assure optimal growth. Inform the selection and type of formula based on the patient nutrition needs and goal of the feeding regimen.

(continued)

**Box 4.5   Roles and Responsibilities of Specialty
                Team Members** (continued)

> • **Nursing**: Provide discharge education to the family on the
>   care and management of the gastrostomy site.
> • **Social work**: Connect the family to resources to provide
>   assistance and support in the home.
> • **Home health agency/insurer**: Delivers the required for-
>   mula and supplies to the family on a regular schedule. In
>   some cases the home health agency will obtain and maintain
>   authorization for equipment and formula. Provides ongoing
>   support in the home.
> • **School (nurse)**: Coordinate information and services when a
>   child requires feeding at school.

WHAT GOES IN THE TUBE?

In general, most pediatric feeding tubes have a small
diameter. Only liquid nutrition is recommended for use
in pediatric feeding tubes. Any food (eg, homemade
blended) or non-food (eg, medications) that could obstruct
or clog the tube must be avoided. For this reason, medications should only be given in liquid form. If medication
in liquid form is not available, then crushed medications
should be administered with a small amount of water as a
flush so as not to interact with formula (1,2). The American Society for Parenteral and Enteral Nutrition (ASPEN)
recommends that the child's age be taken into account
when defining fluid volume for flushing EN tubes with
sterile or purified water. ASPEN also cautions that routine
flushing after each bolus or interrupted continuous feeding in children is *not* recommended. Approximately 3 to 5
mL is typically enough to flush a nasogastric (NG) tube in
children if a tube becomes clogged, with smaller volumes

indicated in premature or smaller infants (2). Medications should not be added to EN, nor should medications be mixed prior to administration (1). Boxes 4.6 and 4.7 identify general categories of enteral formulas (15–18).

Box 4.6   Standard Pediatric Products (1 kcal/mL) Used for Non-oral Feeding

Commercial Cow's Milk–based Formula
- *Benefits:* Most common, readily available; formulated to provide 100% of DRIs in 1,000mL (usually) for children ages 1-10 years.
- *Concerns:* Contains intact cow milk protein. Not indicated for children with cow milk protein allergy. May not be covered by insurance.

Commercial Soy-based Formula
- *Benefits:* Appropriate for vegetarians and children with milk-protein allergies; formulated to provide DRIs in 1,000 mL for children ages 1-10 years.
- *Concerns:* Contains intact soy protein. Not indicated for children with soy protein allergy (10%–14% of children with milk allergy are also allergic to soy).

Commercial Blended (Food) Formula
- *Benefits:* Sterile; made from conventional foods. A complete nutrition product that provides 100% of DRIs in 1,000 mL for children ages 1–20 years.
- *Concerns:* Commercial supplements may not be covered by insurance.

Abbreviation: DRI, Dietary Reference Intake.
Source: Data are from references 15–18.

**Box 4.7   Specialized Pediatric Products Used for
            Non-oral Feeding**

Home Blenderized
- *Benefits:* Allows family to be involved in meal preparation;
  may provide greater nutrient content and variety.
- *Concerns:* Not emulsified; only appropriate delivery is via
  stomach; recommend gastrostomy. May have greater viscos-
  ity and osmolality. May result in delivery of inconsistent
  energy, protein, and other nutrients, and may not meet DRIs.
  Not appropriate for continous feeding due to increased
  potential for bacterial contamination; not sterile.

Calorie-dense (> 1 kcal/mL)
- *Benefits:* Appropriate for children with fluid restriction and/
  or increased metabolic needs.
- *Concerns:* Places children at increased risk for dehydration;
  not recommended for transpyloric feedings.

Semi-elemental
- *Benefits:* Typically indicated for children with
  malabsorption.
- *Concerns:* Expensive, limited palatability for oral feeding.
  Not appropriate for children with allergies to cow's milk and
  soy.

Elemental
- *Benefits:* Appropriate for children with malabsorption and
  severe protein allergy.
- *Concerns:* Expensive; poor palatability for oral feeding;
  higher osmolarity than standard formulas.

Abbreviation: DRI, Dietary Reference Intake.
Source: Data are from references 15–18.

FEEDING SUPPLIES

The use of commercially available complete nutrition supplements, a feeding pump (if indicated), and related supplies, such as bags and tubing, will be required for long-term use. Letters and prescriptions from the child's primary care provider or specialty feeding team for enteral products and feeding supplies are routinely needed for insurance coverage and provision of home health care agency services.

Families sometimes choose to use homemade or blenderized table foods. The use of this type of feeding does introduce serious concerns ranging from inadequate nutrition to bacterial contamination. Even so, many families prefer it as an opportunity to participate in meal preparation (16). It benefits the family because they are involved in the child's meal preparation, and can supply a variety of nutrients while mimicking oral feeding (17). Blenderized feedings are problematic in that caregivers may use uncooked table foods, select foods based on taste rather than nutritional content, underestimate fluid needs, encounter difficulty balancing nutrients and calories, as well as the potential for tube clogging (15,16). Children with low metabolic needs who receive blenderized foods are at increased risk for micronutrient deficiencies, and should be closely monitored through routine anthropometrics and laboratory tests (15). When educating families on the preparation of blenderized feeding, it is critical to stress the importance of food safety (19). Clinical standards that should be met before considering the use of a home blenderized feeding program are listed in Box 4.8 (16).

Box 4.8 Clinical Standards When Considering Home Blenderized Feeding

The *child* must meet the following criteria:
- Be medically stable (no acute changes in health status)
- Have a *gastrostomy* feeding tube greater than 14 French (jejunostomy tubes are never appropriate)
- Be able to tolerate bolus feedings (< 60 minutes).
- Be able to tolerate the volume required to provide optimal nutrition.

The *family* must meet the following criteria:
- Demonstrate interest in providing blenderized food
- Have access to a registered dietitian to monitor tolerance to, and adequacy of, blenderized feeding
- Have access to adequate cooking facilities and hot water
- Have access to a medical grade food blender to assure appropriate consistency
- Have access to adequate storage and refrigeration

Source: Data are from reference 16.

MANAGEMENT OF NON-ORAL FEEDING OR LIMITED ORAL FEEDING

The best intervention for a child who may require nutrition support is to refer him or her to a specialty feeding team (if available), a pediatrician, or a pediatric gastroenterologist. It is especially important to assess the risk of aspiration in children with neurological impairments who may have gastrointestinal dysfunction, such as gastroesophageal reflux disease (GERD) and/or slow gastric emptying (20,21). Keep in mind that once the decision has been made for non-oral feeding, parents accept a great deal of responsibility in the management and delivery of feedings. Box 4.9 outlines some of the key responsibilities that parents will need to assume in providing non-oral feeding to their child.

Box 4.9 Role of the Family in Enteral Nutrition Implementation and Monitoring

- Obtain feeding equipment, supplies, and formula from the home health agency with assistance from a social worker.
- Define the care plan with the interdisciplinary team, reflecting the family and child's needs.
- Maintain a record of the child's growth and keep documentation of any changes in feeding schedule, nutrient intake, and unusual behaviors or tolerance issues exhibited by the child to be shared with the feeding team.
- Identify signs or symptoms that would require the interdisciplinary team or other specialist be contacted for a reevaluation.
- Develop an emergency plan and list of key contacts in the event of an emergency (eg, potential tube feeding complication or illness).
- Attend appointment with community and specialty care providers for ongoing monitoring and care.
- Adjust the schedule and nutritional intake volume as required under the diet prescription as defined by the feeding team.
- Practice optimum safety and sanitation techniques with feeding administration to prevent foodborne illness.

The RD and other members of the specialty feeding team will be called on to support the family as they carry out many of the tasks listed in Box 4.9. Ongoing monitoring is critical to ensure that the infant/child receives adequate nutrition and tolerates feedings; changes in the feeding schedule are made as needed; and parents have adequate supplies as summarized in Table 4.1.

**Table 4.1   Management of Non-Oral Feedings and
the Role of Team Members**

Management of Non-Oral Feedings (Frequency)	Responsible Team Members
Monitor growth and weight gain (3–6 mo; younger children may need to be seen more frequently)	Pediatrician, nurse, registered dietitian (RD)
Assess nutrient adequacy of feeding regimen (3 mo)	RD
Monitor tolerance to feeding (continuously)	Parents, pediatrician, home health nurse, RD, social worker
Adjust feeding schedule[a] (as needed to attain optimal tolerance)	Parent, pediatrician, nurse (in consultation with RD)
Order feeding supplies[b] (monthly)	Social worker, parents/caregivers
Obtain and submit prescriptions for authorization (6–12 mo; may vary by state)	Pediatrician, nurse, health care agency

[a]For example, time and rate.
[b]For example, bags and tubing.

Schedules

After the need for nutrition support has been demonstrated and EN is implemented, the patient must be closely monitored so goals and schedules can be adjusted over time. Box 4.10 provides examples of goals that can be included in nutrition care plans. While some children will require total enteral nutrition, some children may receive partial feeding by mouth with the remaining nutrients delivered non-orally. Using the EN route to deliver medications, meet fluid needs, or use for sick days, may be appropriate for some children. The child's feeding schedule must ensure optimum tolerance and safety. For children receiving continuous drip-feeding via a pump, a daily feeding schedule that is defined by the parent and the specialty feeding team is critical. The feeding schedule should take into account both the child and family's daily schedule, while maintaining an adequate nutrient intake. The length of exposure of the formula to room temperature should be taken into consideration, as hang-times recommended by the manufacturer must be followed to ensure safety (19).

Box 4.10   Examples of Goals and Schedules for Non-oral and Limited Oral Feeding

Example 1
- *Goal:* Weight gain is the primary goal, with a secondary goal of maintaining oral feeding.
- *Sample schedule:* More than half of estimated energy needs are provided at night by pump feedings, and with supplements to meals (lunch, dinner, and snacks) during the day.

Example 2
- *Goal:* Progression of oral feeding skill development is the primary goal, with a secondary goal of weight gain.
- *Sample schedule:* Three meals and two snacks are offered during the day, with bolus feedings delivered after meals (or at night) based on the energy deficit from the day's oral intake.

Example 3
- *Goal:* Recovery from a recent illness and regression of the child's oral feeding skills.
- *Sample schedule:* Up to 80% of total needs provided by continuous drip feedings (at night) and bolus feedings during the day, with oral tastes of favorite foods as much as tolerated.

Example 4
- *Goal:* Transition off gastrostomy feeding is the primary goal, with a secondary goal of weight maintenance (with medical clearance).
- *Sample schedule:* Reduce night feedings by 25%; omit some bolus feedings during the day to allow hunger sensations to emerge; offer meals and snacks at regular intervals. It is critical to individualize transition feeding schedules.

Any oral feeding that is safe should be encouraged for socialization and preservation of oral motor skills. When a return to oral feeding is a long-term goal, daytime bolus feedings without night feedings may make it less likely that this goal can be reached. When developing a feeding schedule, remember that continuous feeding or inadequate spacing between bolus feeds and meals or snacks will lead to decreased oral intake. Inadequate spacing results in decreased hunger and interest in oral feeding over time. Offering food or beverages before bolus feedings may encourage interest in tasting; however, maintaining oral hunger sensations is difficult with closely spaced eating or bolus feeding times. Box 4.11 provides a description of different feeding regimens individualized to meet the needs of the child and his or her family.

Box 4.11 Long-term Gastrostomy Feeding: Examples of Nutrition Plans

Example 1
- *Patient:* 7-year-old girl with spastic quadriplegia and seizures.
- *Nutrition care plan:* Two to three bolus feedings per day and 8-10 hours/night on pump with extra water flushes when medications are given. Provide adequate energy and protein intake from a complete pediatric product, based on child's size and level of activity.

Example 2
- *Patient:* 4-year-old boy with propionic acidemia (an inborn error of metabolism) with age-appropriate eating skills and hospitalizations about two or three times per year.
- *Nutrition care plan:* A low-protein diet of table food and beverages, with contingency feeding of his metabolic formula when his oral intake is less than optimum, when he needs extra fluids, or for formula and medications when ill.

(continued)

**Box 4.11   Long-term Gastrostomy Feeding: Examples of
Nutrition Plans** (continued)

Example 3
- *Patient:* 5-year-old girl with Rett syndrome who is unable to gain weight.
- *Nutrition care plan:* Three meals and two snacks per day fed orally with night gastrostomy feedings for extra energy and nutrients from a complete nutritional supplement.

Example 4
- *Patient:* 8-year-old boy with glycogen storage disease (an inborn error of carbohydrate metabolism) with appropriate oral intake.
- *Nutrition care plan:* Night gastrostomy feeding to prevent hypoglycemia and preserve growth. Regular food and beverages (as allowed) with meals and snacks offered at regular intervals.

Goals for growth and feeding skill progression are individualized to the child. Table 4.2 provides examples of potential problems and trouble-shooting when reassessing the child's nutrition care plan (22). Complications of enteral feedings, such as malabsorption, nausea and vomiting, fever, redness at the feeding site, and other GI issues, should be referred to the primary care provider or gastroenterologist working with the family (7). Box 4.12 provides clinical tips on helping children and their families meeting the established nutrition goals.

Table 4.2 Management of Gastrostomy-Related Problems

Problem	Management Suggestions
Child gains weight rapidly or rate of weight gain is faster than expected for age.	Reduce total amount of EN volume by decreasing rate or number of feedings in order to reduce energy intake while maintaining adequate fluid volume and meeting protein and micronutrient needs.
Child is constipated or has decreased stool volume on a liquid diet.	Switch to a fiber-containing complete nutritional supplement and ensure that adequate fluids are given.
Child retches or vomits during or after feedings.	Offer continuous vs bolus feeding and slow the feeding rate. Regular venting can be helpful before and after EN feeding, daytime feeds maybe better suited than night feeds. In addition, use of an isotonic formula helps alleviate delayed gastric emptying (22).
Parent thinks the child is missing the taste of food; child's mouth is dry.	If swallowing is safe, encourage oral tastes. If swallowing is not safe, wet lips often with glycerin swabs or other acceptable substance.
Gastrostomy site is oozing, inflamed, or uncomfortable.	Routine medical visits are needed to size the device correctly and prevent leakage. Refer to health care team for evaluation of continued discomfort around the wound site.
Child is pulling on device or tubing.	Adjust clothing or netting to cover the abdomen area; do not restrict use of hands.

Box 4.12   Clinical Tips: Helping Families Follow Care Plans

- The goal for the child's eating may change over time because of the family's emotional and coping style, rather than the child's diagnoses. Funding sources can pose limitations that affect the progression of eating or feeding skills. For example, the child's health insurance may pay for a nutritional supplement only if it is delivered via gastrostomy feeding tube. This is often a conundrum when children are able to sustain their weight drinking the formula by mouth but the family cannot afford the supplement without reimbursement. Many insurance companies are willing to cover enteral products as part of a treatment plan. The registered dietitian can work with the family to create a treatment plan that delineates the goals and objectives for treatment.
- If the child is dependent in care and must be lifted and transferred, the family may prefer the child to stay the same weight even if weight gain is recommended. The weight issue may be a sign of their concerns about the future for their child in general. Health professionals should discuss the importance of overall good health and nutritional status for the child, and help the family identify physical and mechanical resources to address lifting and transferring.
- Families of a child who requires nutrition support generally have experienced frustration around oral eating in the past. The assumption that eating is fun and a social activity for the family may not apply. Encourage families to understand that mealtime represents an important opportunity for socialization.
- If a child has a feeding tube (gastrostomy or nasogastric) and is also allowed to eat orally, the nutritional adequacy of the food may not be as important as its texture and consistency in maintaining or progressing oral feeding skills.
- As the child gains weight, the gastrostomy button may need to be changed to a different length or diameter. If the hole is getting bigger, and the device is sized incorrectly, leakage is likely.

Returning to Oral Feeding

Returning to oral feeding after non-oral feeding may or may not be a reasonable goal. It is best to proceed slowly and to balance non-oral and oral intake with other therapeutic and family priorities (4). Box 4.13 lists signs of readiness to return to oral feeding and Table 4.3 defines the roles that team members may perform during the transition. The time required for non-oral to oral feeding transition for each child will require the involvement of school personnel, community service providers, and the formula funders (23). Ideally, the child's nutritional status should stay stable as the transition occurs. Continued involvement of a specialty feeding team is vital, particularly because behavioral consultation may be required. The transition process removes some of the control of feeding from the parents and medical providers and places more control with the child. Often the child will demonstrate increased appetite and oral intake after an illness has passed. This is a sign that the transition has been successful and that EN is no longer necessary.

Box 4.13 Signs of Readiness for a Successful Transition

- Child has interest in oral eating and wants to taste.
- Medical evaluation has ruled out risk of aspiration.
- The family can identify signs of hunger in the child.
- Child is at a healthy weight and could tolerate a small weight loss.
- A transitional feeding plan has been developed with follow-up care identified.
- Family support and their interest in working on oral feeding are ensured.
- A school or therapy program is involved with the plan and has staff with feeding expertise.

Table 4.3 Teamwork in Transition to Oral Feeding

Steps in the Transition Process	Responsible Team Members
Assist family in identifying subtle signs of hunger	All
Develop plan to adjust feeding in order to stimulate hunger	Registered dietitian (RD)
Monitor child's rate of weight gain and growth	Pediatrician, RD
Monitor fluid intake to ensure optimal hydration	Primary care physician, RD, nurse
Possible referral for behavioral support to address food refusal or avoidance (common)	Primary care physician, social work, psychotherapist
Provide meals and snacks at regular intervals	Family, school
Assess oral motor coordination and swallowing safety	Speech or occupational therapist

During the transition period, EN should be delayed approximately one hour prior to the meal to allow hunger sensation and interest in oral feeding. EN should be continued until oral intake is greater than fifty percent of the child's usual nutrient intake for two to three consecutive days. The benefit of providing bolus feedings post-meal include preserving the child's appetite during the meal and allowing the caregiver to alter the amount of EN administered to the child depending on oral intake (24). During transition, it is important that caregivers monitor hydration status and increase water flushes as recommended. The RD plays several key roles in the transition process, such as monitoring growth (weight gain) and ensuring the nutritional adequacy of the diet, while partnering with the family and other health care professionals in developing the plan (25).

CASE STUDY 1: NONAMBULATORY 23-MONTH-OLD BOY

Kevin is a nonambulatory 23-month-old boy with central hypotonia (low muscle tone), who needs feeding re-evaluation.

Findings

Mrs. F, Kevin's mother, expressed frustration stating that he cries and chokes after swallowing only a few bites of oatmeal, grits, or other soft-textured food. She also reports that Kevin can only sit for a short period of time in his high chair before he "slumps" over to one side. Kevin has had multiple upper respiratory illnesses including bronchitis in the last 4 months. Mrs. F also states that Kevin was previously treated for GERD. He has tolerated an increase in his volume of a standard pediatric enteral formula but has not made progress toward accepting food from a spoon. Mrs. F says that according to the pediatrician, Kevin has not gained any weight for 5 months. Mrs. F attributes his poor weight gain to his frequent illnesses.

Recommendations

Reassure the mother that her child is indeed hard to feed, and refer them to a specialty feeding team to evaluate his safety for oral feeding, and optimal positioning during feeding. The evaluation should include a modified barium swallow study or video fluoroscopy to view and assess his swallowing. Depending on the findings of the evaluation consider the use of short-term NG or surgically placed gastrostomy tube (G-tube) or button for feedings to provide nutrition support.

Rationale

Kevin's upper respiratory illnesses may be related to his centralized hypotonia, which can affect swallowing. Poor positioning during feeding can also have a negative impact on the ability to swallow safely. Kevin's underlying neurological disability puts him at elevated risk of aspiration that must be re-evaluated.

CASE STUDY 2: NONAMBULATORY 3-YEAR-OLD GIRL WITH CEREBRAL PALSY

Charisse is a nonambulatory 3-year-old girl with cerebral palsy with hypertonia (high muscle tone) and scoliosis, who needs non-oral feeding support.

Findings

Charisse has experienced a 5% weight loss over the past 3 months. Her body mass index (BMI) and triceps skinfold (TSF) measurement are both below the 5th percentile for age. Charisse's grandmother, Ms. C, reports that she offers Charisse three meals and three snacks per day. Ms. C insists that all of the foods offered are energy- and nutrient-dense foods, "not junk." Ms. C also acknowledges that meals are often stressful and can take more than 45 minutes, even for snacks. Charisse reportedly refuses to eat by pushing the food away and by crying, which can progress to vomiting, about once per week. Other family members have started waking Charisse at night to offer high-calorie supplements. She is more irritable than she used to be. The family is concerned because orthopedic surgery could be scheduled if she were not underweight.

Recommendations

Reassure the family that their child is indeed hard to feed, and refer them to a specialty feeding team for comprehensive feeding evaluation and intervention to correct failure to thrive with failed oral feeding. Consider the use of a gastrostomy feeding tube to support optimal nutrition.

Rationale

There is sufficient evidence to support a finding of undernutrition (TSF < 5th percentile, weight loss, and irritability). Also Charisse expends a lot of energy and focus on eating. If Charisse continues to be exposed to negative feeding experiences, she may stop eating altogether. Surgical intervention for scoliosis requires that Charisse have adequate energy stores (evidenced by TSF) and access to optimal nutrition both pre- and postsurgically.

CASE STUDY 3: NONAMBULATORY 7-YEAR-OLD BOY WITH A GASTROSTOMY TUBE

Sean is a nonambulatory 7-year-old boy who had a gastrostomy tube placed at age 5½ years for failure to thrive and severe oral-motor feeding problems. He has gained weight rapidly in the past year.

Findings

Sean's mother, Ms. B, acknowledges how much easier "everything" has been since Sean received his gastrostomy tube. Sean receives three bolus feedings during the day and 8 hours of continuous drip feedings at night using a standard pediatric nutritional supplement. Ms. B reports that Sean enjoys eating cookies crumbled over ice cream before he goes to bed at night. Sean's personal aide at school reports he eats about one-third of his meal, which is more than the family sees him eat at home.

Sean has gained almost 6 kg and grown about 3 cm in the last 18 months. His BMI and triceps skinfold both rank above the 95th percentile, meaning that he is now obese. Ms. B expressed delight with Sean's weight gain, while his physical therapist expressed the concern that he has outgrown his back brace.

Recommendations

Determine whether the family has been in touch with the specialty providers about his feeding schedule and volume, which need to be adjusted for his current status. Coordinate with the team to prevent further weight gain by decreasing his total energy intake (both daytime bolus and night feedings) and to encourage oral feeding at home and school. The mother is still reacting to her feelings of frustration when Sean was failing to thrive, and she needs support to understand that he may not grow to be as tall as other family members but could instead become overweight.

Rationale

There is sufficient evidence of obesity from his TSF to warrant adjustments in his energy intake by decreasing gastrostomy feedings. Sean's scoliosis may invalidate his BMI. However, his elevated TSF combined with his BMI constitutes evidence of obese status. Sean's ability to progress in his self-feeding skills is encouraging but does not yet predict whether he will be able to maintain a healthy weight on oral feeding alone. The issue of transitioning off gastrostomy feeding could be considered in the future, depending on how much Sean can consume on a consistent basis by mouth.

CASE STUDY 4: NONAMBULATORY 8-YEAR-OLD GIRL WITH CEREBRAL PALSY AND A GASTROSTOMY TUBE

Kelsey is a nonambulatory 8-year-old girl with cerebral palsy who had a gastrostomy tube placed for failure to thrive and severe oral-motor feeding problems when she was 5 years old. Her weight has plateaued over the last year.

Findings

Kelsey has not gained weight in the past 12 months even though the specialty feeding team increased the total volume of her feedings twice over the past 6 months. Her recumbent length has remained unchanged over the past 6 months. Kelsey's TSF measurements have also drifted downward, decreasing from the 50th to 15th percentile. Kelsey is dependent on others for all activities of daily living. Her mother, Ms. M, reports that Kelsey tolerates her feedings with no problems or complications. The family has no problem obtaining the formula. On examination, the gastrostomy site is clean and dry. Ms. M does not consider Kelsey's lack of weight gain a problem and quotes a local physician, who told her all children with cerebral palsy are small.

Recommendations

Determine Kelsey's current intake, based on her reported feeding schedule. Review the health priorities that the family has for Kelsey, including her weight status. Once a good rapport has been established, consider asking whether weight gain would be an acceptable goal. Provide Kelsey's family with information about the impact of poor nutritional status on infection and other indicators of health status. Discuss weight and feeding concerns with the specialty feeding team and primary care provider. Inclusion of a mental health provider on the feeding team may help Kelsey's family express any concerns that they have not felt comfortable discussing in the past. If Kelsey's health status deteriorates related to her nutritional status, other public services may need to be contacted (26).

Rationale

In the absence of any reports of feeding intolerance or increased losses (vomiting or diarrhea), Kelsey should be gaining weight. Families may have unexpressed concerns, about weight management, including day-to-day management issues such as lifting and bathing Kelsey. Once such concerns are identified, community resources to address them can generally be utilized.

REFERENCES

1. Bankhead R, Boullata J, Brantley S, et.al; Board of Directors and Clinical Guidelines Task Force. ASPEN enteral nutrition practice recommendations. *JPEN J Parenter Enteral Nutr.* 2009;33: 122–167.
2. Lyman B, Colombo JM, Gamis JL. Implementation of the plan. In: Corkins MR, ed. *The A.S.P.E.N. Pediatric Nutrition Support Core Curriculum.* Silver Springs, MD: ASPEN; 2010:448–459.
3. Charney P, Malone A. *ADA Pocket Guide to Enteral Nutrition.* Chicago, IL: American Dietetic Association; 2006.
4. Morris SE, Klein MD. *Pre-Feeding Skills: A Resource for Comprehensive Mealtime Development.* 2nd ed. San Antonio, TX: Therapy Skill Builders; 2000.
5. Yang Y, Lucas B, Feucht S. Chapter 10. *Nutrition Interventions for Children with Special Health Care Needs.* 3rd ed. Olympia, WA: Washington State Department of Health; 2010:121–128.
6. Enrione EB, Thomlison B, Rubin A. Medical and psychosocial experiences of family caregivers with children fed enterally at home. *JPEN J Parenter Enteral Nutr.* 2005;29:413–419.

7. Pediatric enteral support. In: Nevin-Folino NL, ed. *Pediatric Manual of Clinical Dietetics.* 2nd ed. Chicago, IL: American Dietetic Association; 2003:471–493.

8. Fung EB, Samson-Fang L, Stallings VA, Conway M, Liptak G, Henderson RC, Worley G, O'Donnell M, Calvert R, Rosenbaum P, Chumlea W, Stevenson RD. Feeding dysfunction is associated with poor growth and health status in children with cerebral palsy. *J Am Diet Assoc.* 2002;102:361–373.

9. Sullivan PB, Bachlet AM, Grant H, Juszczak E, Henry J, Vernon-Roberts A, Warner J, Wells J. Gastrostomy feeding in cerebral palsy: too much of a good thing? *Dev Med Child Neurol.* 2006;48:877–882.

10. Marchand V. Enteral nutrition tube feedings. In: Baker SS, Baker RD, Davis AM. *Pediatric Nutrition Support.* Sudbury, MA: Jones & Bartlett Publishers; 2007:249–259.

11. Pohl JF, Cantrell A. Gastrointestinal and nutritional issues in cerebral palsy. *Pract Gastroenterol.* 2006(May);14–22.

12. Veenker E. Enteral feeding in neurologically impaired children with gastroesophageal reflux: Nissen fundoplication and gastrostomy tube placement versus percutaneous gastrojejunostomy. *J Pediatr Nurs.* 2008;23:400–404.

13. Staiano A. Food refusal in toddlers with chronic diseases. *J Pediatr Gastroenterol Nutr.* 2003;37:225–227.

14. Ekvall SW, Ekvall VK. *Pediatric Nutrition in Chronic Diseases and Developmental Disorders.* New York, NY: Oxford University Press; 2005.

15. Parrish CR. Enteral formula selection: a review of selected product categories. *Pract Gastroenterol.* 2005(June);44–74.

16. Klein MD, Morris SE, *Homemade Blended Formula Handbook.* Tucson, AZ: Mealtime Notions; 2007.

17. Samour PQ, King KH. *Handbook of Pediatric Nutrition.* 3rd ed. Sudbury, MA: Jones and Bartlett Publishers; 2005.

18. Bhatia J, Greer F; Committee on Nutrition. Use of soy protein-based formulas in infant feeding. *Pediatrics.* 2008;121:1062–1068.

19. Robbins ST, Beker LT; Pediatric Nutrition Practice Group. *Infant Feedings: Guidelines for Preparation of Formula and Breastmilk in Health Care Facilities.* Chicago, IL: American Dietetic Association; 2004:90–92.

20. Sandritter T. Gastroesophageal reflux disease in infants and children. *J Pediatr Health Care.* 2003;17:198–205.
21. Batshaw ML, Tuchman M. Nutrition and children with disabilities. In: Batshaw ML, ed. *Children with Disabilities*. 6th ed. Baltimore, MD: Paul H. Brookes; 2007:125–136.
22. Cook R, Blinman T. The case of the wretched retcher. *ICAN: Infant, Child, Adolesc Nutr.* 2009;1:94–97.
23. Schwartz SM, Corredor J, Fisher-Medina J. Diagnosis and treatment of feeding disorders in children with developmental disabilities. *Pediatrics.* 2001;108:671–676.
24. Minard G, Lynsen LK. Enteral access devices. In: American Society for Parenteral and Enteral Nutrition. *The Science and Practice of Nutrition Support: A Case-based Core Curriculum*. Dubuque, IA: Kendall/Hunt Publishing Company; 2001:167–179.
25. Dunitz-Scheer M, Levine A, Roth Y, Kratky E, Beckenbach H, Braegger C, Hauer A, Wilken M, Wittenberg J, Trabi T, Scheer PJ. Prevention and treatment of tube dependency in infancy and early childhood. *ICAN: Infant, Child, Adolesc Nutr.* 2009;1:73–82.
26. Gunther DF, Diekema DS. Attenuating growth in children with profound developmental disability. *Arch Pediatr Adolesc Med.* 2006;160:1013–1017.

Chapter 5

Community Services and Programs

Janet H. Willis, MPH, RD

To support successful nutrition outcomes for children with special health care needs (CSHCN) and their families, it is important to assist each family in accessing nutrition services in their community. When exploring program options, it is helpful to note that eligibility requirements and program benefits may vary from state to state, and certain programs target specific age groups. This chapter provides guidelines for assessing needs and identifying available resources.

IDENTIFYING NEEDS

To determine which resources are appropriate for the child with special needs, begin by identifying the programs in which the family is currently participating and those to which they may be referred for additional nutrition services. Table 5.1 provides a list of key questions to ask parents/guardians about their child's nutrition service needs and access to resources.

Table 5.1   Questions to Identify Nutrition Services and Product Needs

Does Your Child . . .	Ages 0–3 y	Ages 3–5 y	Age > 5 y
	Ask Caregivers of Children		
Receive services from an RD?	X	X	X
Need a special pediatric formula or diet?	X	X	X
Need special feeding equipment (eg, bottles, nipples, spoons, forks, plates)?	X	X	X
Require tube feeding?	X	X	X
Participate in the WIC program?	X	X	
Participate in the Early Head Start program?	X		
Receive therapy services through an early intervention program and have an IFSP?	X		
Participate in the Head Start program?		X	
Receive therapy services through school, and have an IEP or 504 accommodation plan?		X	X
Receive health services through a pediatric specialty clinic, CSHCN program, and/or Medicaid/Medical Assistance program?	X	X	X

Abbreviations: CHSCN, Children with Special Health Care Needs; IEP, individualized education program; IFSP, individualized family service plan; RD, registered dietitian; WIC, Special Supplemental Nutrition Program for Women, Infants, and Children.

WIC REFERRAL CRITERIA

The Special Supplemental Nutrition Program for Women, Infants, and Children (WIC) is a federally funded community nutrition program targeting low-income pregnant and lactating women, as well as infants and young children (up to age 5 years). This program provides supplemental services and food assistance to promote health and nutrition. Many low-income infants and children with special health care needs will qualify for WIC services (1). Contact your client's local health department for specific WIC eligibility requirements, and refer to Box 5.1 for general program information (1). Program benefits may vary from state to state.

Box 5.1 WIC Program Eligibility Criteria and Benefits for Children

Eligibility Criteria (all criteria must be met to receive assistance)
- Low-income Infants and children ≤ age 5 years who reside in the state in which they are applying for WIC. (Income guidelines are based on family size and gross annual income.)
- Nutritional risk factors including low iron levels, elevated serum lead levels, underweight, short stature, failure to thrive, obesity, premature birth or low birth weight, high-risk medical condition, inadequate diet, feeding delays, and environmental risks.

Program Benefits
- Nutrition and health education.
- Nutrition assessments and evaluations.
- Food package, which may be modified for CSHCN if medical documentation is provided (eg, a special formula may be substituted).[a] Children receiving special formula will receive the same child foods with proper documentation.
- Monitoring of immunizations.
- Community referrals.

Abbreviations: CSHCN, children with special health care needs; WIC, Special Supplemental Nutrition Program for Women, Infants, and Children.
[a]Allowances and requirements for modifications may vary from state to state.
Source: Data are from reference 1.

EARLY INTERVENTION PROGRAMS

Early intervention programs are established through Part C of the Individuals with Disabilities Education Act (IDEA) to ensure that infants and toddlers with developmental disabilities have access at an early age to services and support. Early intervention services include interdisciplinary evaluations, care coordination, special therapies for the child, and respite and support services for the family. Registered dietitians (RDs) are considered personnel qualified to provide services for infants and toddlers in the early intervention system. Qualifications for RDs are established by each state based on recommendations from the State Interagency Coordinating Council that provides oversight and sets policies for the service delivery system.

SCHOOL-BASED NUTRITION SERVICES

Many schools participate in the National School Breakfast Program (NSBP) and National School Lunch Program (NSLP), which provides balanced meals for school children. CSHCN should have equal access to these meal programs due to civil rights protections and supporting regulations from the US Department of Agriculture (USDA), which administers these meal programs (2). Based on federal guidelines, school meals are to be modified at no extra charge for a student with disabilities whose medical condition restricts his or her diet and who has a diet prescription on file at the school. These modifications are required for children with disabilities. However, schools may make meal modifications at their discretion for individual children who do not have disabilities but who are medically certified as having a special dietary need (2). School policies should provide guidance for these circumstances.

Public and private schools that do not participate in the USDA-sponsored food and nutrition programs are not required to follow these specific guidelines. However, related legislation such as Section 504 of the Rehabilitation Act of 1973 and the Americans with Disabilities Act require that reasonable accommodations be provided for children with disabilities (2). School policies should provide information on meal modifications in these school settings (3).

The allowable meal modifications following the USDA guidelines for the NSBP and NSLP are described in the following sections. Box 5.2 outlines the information required for a school diet prescription (2–4).

Box 5.2 Components of a School Diet Prescription

- Child's name
- Disability or medical diagnosis with an explanation why it requires a special diet or meal modification
- Description of the major life activity affected by the disability
- Diet prescription:
  - Type of diet: diabetic, reduced/increased calorie, modified texture, etc.
  - List of foods omitted and/or substituted
  - Texture: regular, chopped, ground, pureed
  - Additional information to clarify the diet
- Signature and date by a physician or recognized medical authority

Source: Data are from references 2–4.

School Diet Prescription for a Child with a Disability

Substitutions will be provided for a child with a disability only when supported by a diet prescription signed by a licensed physician (2). A diet prescription form may be requested from the school system. It must include the following components:

- A statement of the child's disability and an explanation of why the disability restricts the diet
- A statement identifying the major life activity affected by the disability
- A list of foods to be omitted from the child's diet and the foods that may be substituted

School Diet Prescription for a Child with a Chronic Condition

For a child who does not have a disability, but who has a chronic medical condition that requires a special diet, a prescription or medical statement must be signed by a recognized medical authority, such as a physician, a physician's assistant, a nurse practitioner, or any other specialist identified by the state education agency (2). This prescription must include the following components:

- A statement identifying the medical or other special need that restricts the child's diet
- A list of foods to be omitted from the child's diet and a list of the foods that may be substituted

Menu Modifications

Diet prescriptions may specify modifications of the school breakfast and lunch menus to accommodate specific children. Tables 5.2 and 5.3 provide potential menu changes for low-calorie and high-calorie diets as well as selected texture modifications (4,5).

Table 5.2   Sample Menu Modifications for School Breakfast

Food	Calorie Modifications	Texture Modifications
Orange juice	• Low-calorie: No change • High-calorie: No change or substitute fruit nectar	• Chopped or ground: No change • Pureed: No change; thicken with applesauce if needed
Oatmeal	• Low-calorie: Serve plain • High-calorie: Add margarine and powdered milk	• Chopped or ground: No change • Pureed: May need to puree with milk, or replace with cream of wheat or grits
Cinnamon roll w/ butter	• Low-calorie: Replace with plain toast • High-calorie: Add margarine	• Chopped: Cut in bite-size pieces • Ground or pureed: Replace with more hot cereal or grits
Milk	• Low-calorie: Low-fat or fat-free • High-calorie: Whole	• Whole, low-fat, or fat-free

Source: Data are from references 4 and 5.

Table 5.3   Sample Menu Modifications for School Lunch

Food	Calorie Modifications	Texture Modifications
Hamburger	• Low-calorie: No change • High-calorie: Add cheese	• Chopped: chop meat • Ground: grind meat, add sour cream • Pureed: puree beef with broth or tomato sauce
Buns	• Low-calorie: Serve plain • High-calorie: Add margarine	• Chopped: Cut in quartered size cubes or substitute noodles • Ground: Substitute rice or chopped noodles • Pureed: Substitute bread crumbs mixed with the pureed beef, or pureed mashed potatoes

(continued)

Table 5.3   Sample Menu Modifications for School Lunch
(continued)

Food	Calorie Modifications	Texture Modifications
French fries	• Low-calorie: Baked potato • High-calorie: No change	• Chopped or ground: Mashed potatoes • Pureed: Puree mashed potatoes and blend with gravy or milk
Broccoli	• Low-calorie: No change • High-calorie: Add margarine or cheese sauce	• Chopped: Well-cooked and chopped • Ground: Well-cooked and mashed • Pureed: Puree with cream soup
Canned peaches	• Low-calorie: No change, if canned in own juice • High-calorie: No change or canned in syrup or peach nectar	• Chopped: Cut in bite-size pieces • Ground: Chopped and mashed • Pureed: Puree with juice or nectar
Milk	• Low-calorie: Low-fat or fat-free • High-calorie: Whole	• Whole, low-fat, or fat-free

Source: Data are from references 4 and 5.

Educational Program Goals and Objectives: Nutrition

The Americans with Disabilities Act of 1990 protects individuals with disabilities from discrimination and provides equal access to programs and services. Likewise, supportive state and federal legislation mandates education and related services for children with disabilities who enroll in public schools. The Individualized Family Service Plan (IFSP), Individualized Education Program (IEP), and the 504 Accommodation Plan are working documents that secure services for CSHCN in educational programs. These plans are developed for children who require specialized services in early intervention and public school–based programs. The IFSP is written for infants and toddlers up to 3 years of age who have developmental disabilities and are being served in early intervention programs. The IEP is designed for preschool and school-aged children with disabilities to provide special education and related services that are appropriate for their learning needs. For school-aged children who are chronically ill and do not require special education services but who have special dietary issues, a 504 Accommodation Plan can be developed. Box 5.3 summarizes the educational programs and planning tools that are available for CSHCN in these settings.

Box 5.3   Educational Programs and Planning Tools for CSHCN

Early Intervention Program
- Serves: Infants and toddlers birth to 3 years with developmental disabilities.
- Criteria: Infants and toddlers who have a demonstrated delay in at least one of the following areas: cognitive, physical, communication, social/emotional development, and self-help or adaptive skills; or at the discretion of the state have a diagnosed condition that puts the child at high risk for developmental delays. Examples include seizure disorder, intraventricular hemorrhage, fetal alcohol syndrome, spina bifida, congenital or acquired hearing loss, visual impairment, genetic disorder, brain or spinal cord trauma, inborn errors of metabolism, microcephaly, failure to thrive, and symptomatic congenital infection.
- Planning tool: IFSP.

(continued)

Box 5.3   Educational Programs and Planning Tools for CSHCN
(continued)

Public School (Special Education)
- Serves: School-age children receiving special education services.
- Criteria: Children with physical or intellectual disabilities that substantially limit one or more major life activity. Examples include autism, deaf-blindness, deafness, developmental delay, emotional disturbance, hearing impairment, intellectual disability, multiple disabilities, orthopedic impairment, specific learning disability, speech and language impairment, traumatic brain injury, and visual impairment.
- Planning tool: IEP.

Public School (Regular Education)
- Serves: School-age children with chronic conditions who do not require special education services.
- Criteria: Children with chronic conditions that may require health-related services, but do not require special education services. Examples may include chronic renal disease, controlled seizure disorder, cystic fibrosis, diabetes, hemophilia, and juvenile arthritis.
- Planning tool: 504 Accommodation Plan.

Abbreviations: CSHCN, children with special health care needs; IEP, Individualized Education Program; IFSP, Individualized Family Service Plan.

Individualized plans include annual goals or outcomes, short-term objectives, and a schedule for evaluation. Parents, therapists, and staff are involved in the planning process to ensure that appropriate goals and objectives are identified and monitored for each child. Each goal and objective should be measurable so that the child's progress can be assessed within a designated time period. Incorporating nutrition goals and objectives into these plans will facilitate the delivery of services to improve the nutritional status of CSHCN (4,6,7). Box 5.4 provides an outline of program considerations for developing nutrition-related goals and objectives for an IFSP, IEP, or 504 Accommodation Plan (6). Examples of goals and objectives are provided in Boxes 5.5, 5.6, and 5.7. Boxes 5.8 and 5.9 provide clinical tips related to early interventions and working with schools, children, and caregivers to facilitate nutrition goals.

**Box 5.4   Nutrition Goals and Program Considerations for an
                    IFSP, IEP, or 504 Accommodation Plan**

Nutrition Goals
- Develop or refine self-feeding skills.
- Improve mealtime behavior.
- Communicate nutrition needs such as hunger or thirst.
- Improve growth.
- Improve quality of diet.

Program Considerations
- Identify special feeding equipment and measuring equipment for tracking growth.
- Identify supervision needed for mealtime.
- Identify positive reinforcements Identify personnel responsible for specific tasks such as tracking weight and growth measurements, providing scheduled snacks, monitoring progress on specific goals, etc.
- Provide training for staff.

Source: Adapted with permission from Horsley JW, Allen ER, Daniel PW. *Nutrition Management of School Age Children With Special Needs: A Resource Manual for School Personnel, Families, and Health Professionals.* 2nd ed. Richmond, VA: Virginia Department of Education and Virginia Department of Health; 1996.

Box 5.5 Sample Early Intervention Program Nutrition Plan

- **Patient**: JW, a 20-month-old boy with Down syndrome and developmental delays, receives physical therapy, occupational therapy, and nutrition services through the local early intervention program. He drinks fluids from a bottle and eats strained baby foods three times per day. In addition to his delayed feeding skills, he eats only a limited variety of foods. His weight gain and growth, as well as the quality of his diet are monitored by the registered dietitian (RD). He has an Individualized Family Service Plan (IFSP) that includes a nutrition component.
- **IFSP nutrition goal/outcome**: JW will demonstrate improved feeding skills.
- **IFSP nutrition objectives**:
  - JW will practice cup-drinking skills at one meal, 5 days per week for the next 3 months.
  - JW will try at least one new food each week at home for 6 months.
  - JW will progress to eating pureed foods without resistance within 6 months.

Box 5.6 Sample School Nutrition Plan in Special Education

- **Patient**: SH, a 7-year-old girl with spastic cerebral palsy and a seizure disorder, is extremely underweight and has delayed feeding skills. Her lunch is pureed and an aide feeds her at mealtime. Her Individualized Education Program (IEP) includes a nutrition component to address her need for weight gain.
- **IEP nutrition goal**: SH will eat a high-calorie diet of a pureed consistency at school to support her weight and growth.
- **IEP nutrition objectives**:
  - SH will drink 4 ounces of an energy-dense/high-protein supplement with her school breakfast 75% of the time.
  - SH will eat a school lunch supplemented with energy-dense additives (eg, margarine, powdered milk, cheese sauces, gravy) 75% of the time.

Box 5.7   **Sample School Nutrition Plan for a 504 Accommodation Plan**

- **Patient**: BJ, a 9-year-old boy with type 1 diabetes mellitus, is in a regular education program with a 504 Accommodation Plan for his diabetes. He receives insulin injections, and his physician has prescribed a diabetic diet that is composed of three meals and three snacks daily. BJ is growing well. He needs supervision to ensure that he eats his snacks on a regular schedule to prevent episodes of hypoglycemia.
- **504 Plan nutrition goal**: BJ will maintain blood glucose levels within normal limits.
- **504 Plan nutrition objectives**:
  - BJ will eat a snack at 10 AM and 2 PM on at least four out of five days at school.
  - BJ will report his blood glucose levels to the school nurse every Friday morning with 90% compliance.

Box 5.8   **Clinical Tips: Effective Interactions with Early Intervention Services**

- When referring an infant or toddler to early intervention services, there must be a documented disability, a demonstrated delay in one or more domains (eg, cognitive, developmental, speech, motor, psychosocial, or self-help skills), or a diagnosis of a physical or intellectual condition that puts the child at high risk for developmental delays (refer to Box 5.3). Infants and children with special health needs may have feeding problems or altered energy needs that lead to failure to thrive. For example, these feeding problems are often identified in premature and low-birth-weight infants, and in young children with bronchopulmonary dysplasia, cerebral palsy, or Down syndrome. Failure to thrive is considered a physical condition that puts a child at risk for developmental delays and may provide a basis for enrollment in early intervention services. However, other nutritional deficits and growth delays are often difficult to quantify as part of the eligibility criteria for early intervention. To identify a child eligible for services, other health care providers or therapists

(continued)

**Box 5.8   Clinical Tips: Effective Interactions with Early
Intervention Services** (continued)

> may need to determine percent delays in one or more of the
> mentioned domains. In some states, the referral can be made
> for a suspected delay and the finding agency then makes the
> decision regarding the child's eligibility. Once enrolled in
> the early intervention services, a young child with significant
> nutrition and growth issues may benefit from having a nutri-
> tion care plan that is integrated into the IFSP.
> • When early intervention programs do not have a registered
> dietitian (RD) as part of their interdisciplinary team, they
> should be able to assist with a referral in the community.
> RDs serving CSHCN may be found in a local hospital,
> health department, or University Center for Excellence in
> Developmental Disabilities (UCEDDs; formerly university-
> affiliated programs), or through the local dietetic association.

**Box 5.9   Clinical Tips: Working with Caregivers, Children,
and Schools**

> • Work with parents/guardians to secure nutrition services
> in schools and early intervention programs by requesting a
> nutrition plan in the IFSP, IEP, or 504 Accommodation Plan.
> Encourage parents to request these additions to the plan and
> be available to provide consultation to the planning team.
> • If you are working with a school-age child who requires
> a special diet, ask about the child's participation in school
> breakfast and lunch programs. Provide parents/guardians
> with a diet prescription if a menu modification or food sub-
> stitution is required and contact the school nutrition program
> manager at the school to offer consultation.
> • If a child requires a snack as part of his or her meal plan at
> school, it must be scheduled with the school. Snacks are not
> considered part of the standard school meal plan and are not
> provided by the Child Nutrition Program or other school
> program unless they are specified in the IEP or 504 Plan.
> Some families may decide to send snacks to school for their
> children.
>
> (continued)

**Box 5.9   Clinical Tips: Working with Caregivers, Children,
and Schools** (continued)

- If a child has severe food allergies resulting in life-
  threatening reactions, documentation by a licensed physician
  is needed for schools to make food substitutions. In this
  circumstance, the food allergy is treated as a disability and
  a diet prescription is required.
- In addition to making provisions for meal modifications,
  continue to educate children about their nutrition so that they
  can learn to make healthy food choices. Encourage older
  children and adolescents to take responsibility for their diet
  and food choices.
- To address complex feeding problems in infants and children, work with an interdisciplinary feeding team.

REIMBURSEMENT AND FINANCIAL ASSISTANCE FOR NUTRITION SERVICES AND PRODUCTS

When developing the nutrition care plan for a CSHCN, it
will be important to clarify reimbursement issues related
to the following:

- Nutrition follow-up services
- Pediatric formula, supplements, and modular
  products
- Special feeding equipment (ie, special nipples,
  bottles, spoons, cups, plates, etc)
- Tube feeding equipment (ie, feeding tubes, pumps,
  and supplies)

The following sections identify selected resources
that may help with reimbursement or provide assistance
in obtaining formula, supplies, and/or equipment. Note
that eligibility criteria and program benefits for these

programs can vary from state to state. Information may be obtained by contacting the programs in a locality, or checking the Web site for the state program. For referral information, contact the local health department, school district, or department of social services in the community. Certain programs will provide basic nutrition services and nutrition education but not medical nutrition therapy (MNT), so families should inquire about the type of service when seeking information. (For a summary table of these resources, subscribe to the online version of this pocket guide.)

Early Intervention (EI) Programs

RDs who meet the minimum training criteria as specified by the Interagency Coordinating Council are qualified to provide or supervise EI services. They may be part of an EI team or hired as consultants. Families may need a denial from their insurance company prior to receiving nutrition services.

EI programs may be the payer of last resort for pediatric formula, metabolic formulas and tube feeding supplies or special feeding equipment, particularly if it is specified in the IFSP.

Head Start and Early Head Start

Certain programs may have an RD or nutrition consultant. The focus is on nutrition education rather than MNT or specialized nutrition services. For pediatric, tube feeding, or metabolic formula coverage, a child must have a diet prescription on file with the meal modification, substitutions, or additions, including the special formula needs. These programs do not provide reimbursement for tube feeding supplies or special feeding equipment.

Indian Health Services (IHS)

Each Tribal Program makes decisions regarding their local health programs. IHS inpatients receive nutrition and dietary services while in the hospital. Upon discharge other community resources such as WIC or Head Start may be utilized.

IHS programs do not provide reimbursement for pediatric formula or tube feeding products; metabolic formula for treatment of inborn error of metabolism; tube feeding supplies; or special feeding equipment.

Medicaid/Early Periodic Screening, Diagnosis, and Treatment (EPSDT)

EPSDT may potentially pay for nutrition services. The program has strict criteria for providers and the number of visits. This may be a resource for families for pediatric, tube feeding and metabolic formulas, as well as tube feeding supplies and special feeding equipment.

Formula Manufacturers and Charitable Organizations

Emergency supplies of pediatric, tube feeding or metabolic formula may be available on a case-by-case basis for a family in need. Special bottles and nipples are available from certain companies for cleft lip/palate and neonatal units or nurseries.

Private Insurance

Reimbursement for formulas, supplies, equipment, and nutrition services varies by plan. The RD must have a provider number to bill for services. For more information, check with your state MNT reimbursement representative through the state dietetic association.

State Children's Health Insurance Program (SCHIP)

SCHIP may potentially pay for nutrition services and special feeding equipment. Criteria for pediatric, tube feeding, and metabolic formulas vary by state. SCHIP is a potential resource for tube feeding and special feeding equipment.

State Title V Program: Children with Special Health Care Needs (CSHCN) Program

CSHCN programs may be a potential source for nutrition services or may help pay for such services. These programs may also pay for pediatric, tube feeding, or metabolic formula for eligible children and for tube feeding and special feeding equipment.

Supplemental Security Income (SSI)

Monthly cash payments from SSI may be used to pay for nutrition services; pediatric, tube feeding, or metabolic formula; or tube feeding and special feeding equipment. **Note**: SSI eligibility may also assist a child to be eligible for Medicaid as another resource for nutrition services, products, or equipment.

TRICARE

TRICARE (formerly CHAMPUS) is insurance for military families and may be a potential payment mechanism for medically necessary nutrition services; pediatric, tube feeding, or metabolic formula; or tube feeding and special feeding equipment for eligible families.

Food Stamps (USDA)

Certain associated programs may provide general nutrition education related to the use of food stamps. Food stamps may be used to purchase pediatric, tube feeding, or metabolic formula that is nutritionally complete. They may not be used for tube feeding supplies or special feeding equipment.

NSBP and NSLP (USDA)

For nutrition services, usually a referral is made to a community resource. A diet prescription must either be on file at school for meal modifications, substitutions and additions, including special formulas; or specific diet needs must be stated in the IEP or 504 Accommodation Plan.

Special feeding equipment may be covered if it is included in the child's IEP. Otherwise, a school therapist may make inexpensive adaptive feeding equipment on a case-by-case basis.

WIC (USDA)

A nutrition screening/evaluation is a required component of the WIC program. Pediatric, tube feeding, and metabolic formulas may be provided by prescription. Selection may be limited due to state contracts with suppliers. Quantity is limited. WIC does not provide or pay for tube feeding supplies or special feeding equipment.

PARENT ADVOCACY AND SUPPORT GROUPS

In addition to offering emotional support, parent support groups and advocacy groups can help families with CSHCN gather information and navigate the service system. The local telephone directory, library, and neighborhood newspapers are generally good sources for locating a specific group. The Internet is a resource for finding information and locating other families of children with rare syndromes and disorders. Families and providers should be cautioned that nutrition misinformation and financial frauds may be mixed with credible information on the Internet and by local groups, so it is important to carefully review information and ask questions to validate the reliability of claims. Recommending groups for psychosocial support and encouraging parents to ask questions or bring materials to clinic appointments may help families obtain accurate information. See Box 5.10 for additional clinical tips related to building effective partnerships with families.

Box 5.10   Clinical Tips: Creating Successful Partnerships with Families

- Partner with families in decision-making about the services and support systems appropriate for their child. Be open to family views and respectful of the family culture.
- Encourage families to discuss their concerns, questions, and ideas for treatments. Often parents are reluctant to report alternative treatments that they are trying. Encourage an open discussion in order to share information about alternative therapies, reinforce helpful and safe strategies, and discourage unsafe practices.
- Remember to encourage grandparents, extended family members, and other caregivers to participate in support and advocacy groups. Sibling groups are also available in certain communities and can provide needed supports for brothers and sisters of children with special health care needs.

INTERNET RESOURCES

To learn about programs from a national perspective, the Web sites listed in Box 5.10 may be useful. Keep in mind that there is variability in program criteria and benefits in every state.

Box 5.11 Web Sites for National Services and Programs

- **Title V CSHCN Program**: http://mchb.hrsa.gov/programs/titlevgrants/index.html
- **US Department of Agriculture Food and Nutrition Information Service** (National School Breakfast and Lunch Programs; the Special Supplemental Nutrition Program for Women, Infants, and Children [WIC]; and Food Stamps Program): www.fns.usda.gov/fns
- **Individuals with Disabilities Education Act (IDEA)**, including early intervention and special education services:
  - National Early Childhood Technical Assistance Center: http://nectac.org/partc/partc.asp#overview
  - National Dissemination Center for Children with Disabilities—Babies and Toddlers: www.nichcy.org/BABIES/Pages/Default.aspx
  - National Dissemination Center for Children with Disabilities—Children: www.nichcy.org/EducateChildren/Pages/Default.aspx
- **Medicaid**: www.cms.gov/home/medicaid.asp
- **State Children's Health Insurance Program** (SCHIP):
  - Centers for Medicare & Medicaid Services: www.cms.hhs.gov/home/chip.asp
  - Insure Kids Now Web site: www.insurekidsnow.gov
- **Supplemental Security Income (SSI)—Benefits for Children with Disabilities**: www.ssa.gov/pubs/10026.html
- **Indian Health Services**: http://www.ihs.gov

CASE STUDY 1: PREMATURELY BORN TODDLER GIRL WITH POOR GROWTH

MG is a 22-month-old girl who was born prematurely and her family is new to the community. As a toddler with growth failure, she requires special pediatric formula.

Findings

MG was born 2 months premature with bronchopulmonary dysplasia (BPD). Her chronological age is 22 months and her corrected age is 20 months. Each day she drinks approximately 26 oz of 24 kcal/oz infant formula from a bottle. Her mother also feeds her three meals of soft table foods and some stage 2 meats. In the last 6 months, MG has lost 2 lb and her length is stable. She is the only child in a low-income family that is new to the community and has few resources. She is enrolled in an early intervention program because of delays in the areas of speech and fine- and gross-motor skills. MG will receive weekly home-based therapy services. The staff is concerned with her lack of growth and recognizes the need for a nutrition assessment, but an RD is not a part of the program.

Recommendations

- Refer family to Medicaid and Title V/CSHCN programs for medical services.
- Refer family to WIC program for nutrition services and a specialized food package. If a more in-depth nutrition assessment is needed, the Title V/CSHCN program may have an RD on staff or on a referral network who can complete a nutrition evaluation. Additional resources may include a local neonatal intensive care unit (NICU) follow-up clinic or a pediatric RD at a local hospital.
- Develop a plan, monitor progress, and make other appropriate referrals.
- Recommend a complete commercial pediatric formula that provides 30 kcal/oz as part of the WIC food package. Obtain a prescription for the formula from the primary care physician.

- Request care coordination from the early intervention program to assist the family in coordinating appointments.
- Consult with the RD to whom she was referred to develop nutrition goals/outcomes and objectives for the IFSP.

Rationale

A variety of resources is available for low-income CSHCN. Early intervention programs provide care coordination for families and can assist with the referral process for needed services. All programs need to be coordinated to provide continuity of care. The IFSP is an excellent tool to assist families and providers to target goals for a child and to monitor progress. The pediatric nutrition formula will provide increased energy and protein intake without increasing the volume of intake.

CASE STUDY 2: OVERWEIGHT SCHOOL-AGE BOY WITH SPINA BIFIDA AND LEARNING DISABILITIES

GM is an 8-year-old boy with spina bifida and learning disabilities. He is overweight, receives special education services, and requires diet modifications and new equipment.

Findings

GM is enrolled in the second grade and receives special education services in his local public school. He has gained 10 lb in the last 6 months, has short stature, and has outgrown his wheelchair. GM participates in the school breakfast and lunch programs. He receives care from an RD in the regional spina bifida specialty clinic and has Medicaid benefits.

Recommendations

- Design a balanced low-calorie diet for weight main-tenance and continued linear growth with input from the child and family. Discuss this diet plan with the RD in the spina bifida clinic.
- Contact the primary care provider to obtain a diet prescription for the school. Discuss plans for the diet with the family and school nutrition program manager. Recommend that the IEP include goals regarding dietary modifications and increased activity level through an adaptive physical education program.
- Refer to physical therapy for evaluation of GM's wheelchair and for processing of paperwork for wheelchair revisions through Medicaid, as well as recommendations for physical activity at school and at home.
- Follow-up in 1 month to monitor progress and adjust the plan as needed.

Rationale

The goal of weight maintenance is appropriate for a growing school-age child who is overweight. Children with spina bifida usually have a low metabolic rate and need calorie-controlled diets to prevent obesity. Their diets must be planned so that the energy restrictions do not interfere with linear growth. For the best outcome, the meal modifications and activity schedule should be coordinated between the home and school. The IEP is a planning tool to facilitate a coordinated plan. Specialty clinics provide comprehensive care for CSHCN. Some clinics have RDs on staff, and others may make referrals for nutrition services.

CASE STUDY 3: INFANT GIRL WITH PHENYLKETONURIA WHO IS IN NEED OF FINANCIAL ASSISTANCE

ML is a 1-month-old girl who has phenylketonuria (PKU). As an infant with inborn error of metabolism, she requires a special metabolic formula but her family's insurance will not pay for the product.

Findings

ML was diagnosed with PKU shortly after birth through a newborn screening program. Her family's income is more than the income level for Medicaid and WIC services. ML was initially evaluated through the state metabolic treatment program, which is located 1 hour away from her home. She receives follow-up and routine medical exams from her primary care physician in her community.

Recommendations

- Contact the formula manufacturer for an initial emergency supply of the formula until other arrangements can be made.
- Enroll family in the state metabolic treatment program through the Title V program in the state health department, which coordinates treatment, medical nutrition therapy by an RD, and assistance with obtaining the formula.

Rationale

The metabolic formula is necessary to control phenylalanine levels and prevent intellectual disability and other medical complications. Metabolic formula is used in combination with either breastmilk or a regular commercial formula that will provide an amount of phenylalanine to meet the infant's essential needs. In many states, the metabolic treatment program will provide assistance for families through a sliding fee scale based on family income. WIC programs may be a source for metabolic formula if financial criteria are met. The treatment program can provide periodic evaluations and consultations with the local physician. This program is available through the Title V program in the state health department.

CASE STUDY 4: SCHOOL-AGE GIRL WITH CYSTIC FIBROSIS

KT is a 7-year-old girl with cystic fibrosis (CF). Because she has a chronic disease, she requires a special diet and support services at school.

Findings

KT is underweight and has lost 4 lb in the past 2 months. She is hungry constantly and eats well at school. KT participates in the school breakfast and lunch programs. She complains about stomach cramps and uses the bathroom frequently. She is self-conscious about taking her enzymes and will often neglect to take them at school. KT is followed by a medical team, including an RD, through a CF center at the university medical center. When the team reevaluated her, they developed the following recommendations.

Recommendations

- Reinforce for KT and her family the need for enzyme replacement therapy with meals and snacks.
- Design a meal plan with KT and her family that includes three high-calorie meals and two snacks daily.

- Have parents request a 504 Accommodation Plan that includes a high-calorie diet, scheduled snacks, and monitoring of KT's intake of enzymes. This will reinforce her treatment program at school as well as at home.
- Provide a diet prescription for a high-calorie diet and scheduled snacks at school. Coordinate the plan with the school nutrition program manager.
- Consider counseling for KT to help her with her feelings of self-consciousness.

Rationale

Individuals with CF have insufficient levels of pancreatic enzymes to digest and absorb most fats, proteins, and some carbohydrates. Enzyme replacement therapy is necessary to prevent malabsorption. Children with CF require increased energy intake for their age to meet their high metabolic needs and support growth. The 504 Plan is a tool for securing health-related services for students with chronic conditions who are not served in special education programs. Parents and school personnel contribute to the success of the treatment plan.

SUMMARY

Children with special health care needs are at increased risk of encountering difficulties for community services. To promote successful growth and health, families and medical teams should be observant of the child's needs and available local and national resources. When programs become stressful as a result of battling, the child's health may be at risk and professional assistance should be sought to assess the situation. Difficulties do not have to consume the daily life of the child and or family members, and can be managed with the support of interdisciplinary team members.

REFERENCES

1. US Department of Agriculture Food and Nutrition Service. WIC Program. http://www.fns.usda.gov/wic. Accessed February 18, 2011.

2. US Department of Agriculture, Food and Nutrition Service. *Accommodating Children with Special Dietary Needs in School Nutrition Programs: Guidance for School Food Service Staff.* 2001. http://www.fns.usda.gov/cnd/guidance/special_dietary_needs.pdf. Accessed February 18, 2011.

3. Medlen JEG. *The Down Syndrome Nutrition Handbook: A Guide to Promoting Healthy Lifestyles.* Portland, OR: Phronesis Publishing; 2006.

4. *CARE: Special Nutrition for Kids.* Rev ed. Montgomery, AL: Alabama State Department of Education, Child Nutrition Programs; 1995.

5. National Dysphagia Diet Task Force. *National Dysphagia Diet: Standardization for Optimal Care.* Chicago IL: American Dietetic Association; 2002.

6. Horsley JW, Allen ER, Daniel PW. *Nutrition Management of School Age Children with Special Needs: A Resource Manual for School Personnel, Families, and Health Professionals.* 2nd ed. Richmond, VA: Virginia Department of Education and Virginia Department of Health; 1996.

7. Willis, JH, Shockey WL. Serving children with special needs. In: Martin MJ, Oakley CB, eds. *Managing Child Nutrition Programs: Leadership for Excellence.* 2nd ed. Sudbury, MA: Jones and Bartlett Publishers; 2008:445–475.

Resources

BOOKS, MANUALS, MODULES, AND NEWSLETTERS ON SPECIAL HEALTH CARE NEEDS

Baker SS, Baker RD, Davis AM. *Pediatric Nutrition Support*. Jones & Bartlett Publishers; 2007.

Cloud HH, Bomba A, Carithers T, Tidwell D. *Handbook for Children with Special Food and Nutrition Needs*. National Food Service Management Institute; 2006. www.nfsmi.org/documentLibrary Files/PDF/20080213015556.pdf.

Cox JH. *Nutrition Manual for At-Risk Infants and Toddlers*. Precept Press; 1997. Ekvall SW, Ekvall VK. *Pediatric Nutrition in Chronic Diseases and Developmental Disorders*. 2nd ed. Oxford University Press; 2005.

Groh-Wargo S, et al. *Nutritional Care for High-Risk Newborns*. Revised 3rd ed. Precept Press; 2000.

Guralnick MJ, ed. *Interdisciplinary Clinical Assessment of Young Children with Developmental Disabilities*. Brookes Publishing; 2000. www.brookespublishing.com.

Klein MD, Delany T. *Feeding and Nutrition for the Child with Special Needs: Handouts for Parents*. Therapy Skill Builders; 1994. www.pearsonassessments.com.

Medlin JG. *The Down Syndrome Nutrition Handbook—A Guide to Promoting Healthy Lifestyles*. Phronesis Publishing; 2002. www.DownSyndromeNutrition.com

Morris S, Klein M. *Pre-Feeding Skills: A Comprehensive Resource for Feeding Development*. 2nd ed. Therapy Skill Builders; 2000. www.pearsonassessments.com.

National Food Service Management Institute. *CARE Connection: Special Needs in Child Care*. 2011. http://nfsmi-web01.nfsmi .olemiss.edu/ResourceOverview.aspx?ID=275.

Nutrition Focus for Children with Special Health Care Needs (newsletter published six times annually, with each issue focused on a specific disorder or condition). http://depts.washington.edu/ chdd/ucedd/ctu_5/nutritionnews_5.html.

Nutrition Strategies for Children with Special Needs. 2nd ed. UAP Center for Child Development and Developmental Disabilities, Children's Hospital Los Angeles; 2005. www.uscucedd.org/index.php?option=com_content&view=article&id=166&Itemid=230 or 323/669-5948.

Ogata B, et al. *Nutrition for Children with Special Health Care Needs* (Web-based modules). Pacific West MCH Distance Learning Network; 2002. http://depts.washington.edu/pwdlearn.

Pediatric Nutrition Practice Group. *ADA Pocket Guide to Neonatal Nutrition.* American Dietetic Association; 2009. www.eatright.org/shop.

Pediatric Nutrition Practice Group. *Infant Feedings: Guidelines for the Preparation of Human Milk and Formula in Health Care Facilities.* 2nd ed. Pediatric Nutrition Practice Group. American Dietetic Association; 2011. www.eatright.org/shop.

Project Chance: A Guide to Feeding Young Children with Special Needs. Arizona Department of Health Services, Office of Nutrition Services; 1995. http://clas.uiuc.edu/fulltext/cl02220/cl02220.html.

Pronsky ZM, Crowe JP, Elbe D, Young VSL. *Food Medication Interactions.* 16th ed. Food Medication Interactions; 2010.

Tluczek A, Sondel S. *Project SPOON: Special Program of Oral Nutrition for Children with Special Needs.* 1991. HRSA Information Center item code MCHE016. www.ask.hrsa.gov.

Wolf LS, Glass RP. *Feeding and Swallowing Disorders in Infancy: Assessment and Management.* Pearson Education; 1992. www.pearsonassessments.com.

Yang Y, Lucas B, Feucht S, eds. *Nutrition Interventions for Children with Special Health Care Needs.* 3rd ed (free download). Washington State Department of Health; 2010. http://here.doh.wa.gov/materials/nutrition-interventions/15_CSHCN-NI_E10L.pdf.

BOOKS, MANUALS, MODULES, AND NEWSLETTERS ON GENERAL PEDIATRIC NUTRITION

Academy of Nutrition and Dietetics. Pediatric Nutrition Care Manual. Updated annually. www.peds.nutritioncaremanual.org.

Hendricks KM, Duggan C. *Manual of Pediatric Nutrition.* 4th ed. BC Decker; 2005.

Kleinman RE. *Pediatric Nutrition Handbook*. 6th ed. Elk Grove, IL: American Academy of Pediatrics; 2008.

Leonberg B. *ADA Pocket Guide to Pediatric Nutrition Assessment*. American Dietetic Association; 2008. www.eatright.org/shop.

Samour PQ, et al. *Pediatric Nutrition*. 4th ed. Jones and Bartlett Learning; 2010. www.jbpub.com.

NUTRITION-RELATED WEB SITES

Assuring Pediatric Nutrition in the Community. General guidelines, frequently asked questions, resources, continuing education, training opportunities. http://depts.washington.edu/nutrpeds.

CDC Growth Charts. www.cdc.gov/growthcharts. Training materials available at: http://depts.washington.edu/growth.

Dietary Reference Intakes. Institute of Medicine, National Academies Press. www.nap.edu.

Gaining and Growing. Focus on nutrition follow-up of premature infants in the community. https://staff.washington.edu/growing.

Nutrition Services for Children with Special Health Care Needs in Washington State. Information for health care providers and families (general and Washington State), including links to reimbursement reports and other resources. http://depts.washington.edu/cshcnnut.

US Department of Agriculture. Includes the National School Breakfast and Lunch Programs, the Supplemental Nutrition Program for Women, Infants, and Children [WIC], and Food Stamps Program. www.fns.usda.gov/fns.

WEB SITES FOR FOOD AND NUTRITION PROFESSIONALS

Behavioral Health Nutrition. A dietetic practice group of the Academy of Nutrition and Dietetics. www.bhndpg.org.

Pediatric Nutrition Practice Group. A dietetic practice group of the Academy of Nutrition and Dietetics. www.pediatricnutrition.org.

Self-study Curriculum: Nutrition for Children with Special Health Care Needs. 2008. Pacific West Distance Learning

Network. This continuing education activity is designed for registered dietitians and other health care professionals who see children with special health care needs as part of their clinical practices. http://depts.washington.edu/pwdlearn/web.

WEB SITES RELATED TO MEDICAL, EDUCATIONAL, FINANCIAL, AND SUPPORTIVE SERVICES

American Association on Mental Retardation. Professional association promoting policies, research, effective practices, and universal human rights for people with intellectual disabilities. www.aamr.org.

Exceptional Parent Magazine. Information, support, ideas, and outreach for parents and families of children with disabilities and the professionals who work with them. www.eparent.com.

Families and Advocates Partnership for Education (FAPE). Information about Individuals with Disabilities Education Act (IDEA). www.fape.org/idea/index.htm.

Family Village. A global community that integrates information, resources, and communication opportunities on the Internet for persons with cognitive and other disabilities, their families, and service providers. www.familyvillage.wisc.edu.

Family Voices. Partnering with professionals and families to advocate for health care services that are family-centered, community-based, comprehensive, coordinated, and culturally competent. www.familyvoices.org.

Federal Interagency Coordinating Council. Established by IDEA legislation serving young children with disabilities; provides links to state interagency coordinating councils. www.fed-icc .org.

Federation for Children with Special Needs. www.fcsn.org.

Food Allergy and Anaphylaxis Network (FAAN). Support, education and advocacy for those living with food allergies and sensitivities. Publishes *Food Allergy News* six times a year. www .foodallergy.org.

Genetic Alliance. Support, education, and advocacy for those living with genetic conditions. www.geneticalliance.org.

IDEA Partnership. Collaboration of more than 50 national organizations, technical assistance providers, and organizations and agencies at state and local level. Together with the Office of

Special Education Programs (OSEP), the partner organizations aim to improve outcomes for students and youth with disabilities. http://www.ideapartnership.org.

Indian Health Services, US Department of Health and Human Services. www.ihs.gov.

Maternal and Child Health Bureau, Health Resources and Services Administration, US Department of Health and Human Services Title V Maternal and Child Health Services Block Grant Program. http://mchb.hrsa.gov/programs/titlevgrants/index.html.

Medicaid Program, Centers for Medicare & Medicaid Services, US Department of Health and Human Services. www.cms.gov/home/medicaid.asp.

National Down Syndrome Society. A comprehensive resource for Down syndrome. http://www.ndss.org.

National Early Childhood Technical Assistance Center. Information on Individuals with Disabilities Education Act (IDEA). http://nectac.org/partc/partc.asp#overview.

National Information Center for Children and Youth with Disabilities. Targeted mainly toward educational programs. www.NICHCY.org.

National Organization for Rare Diseases (NORD). www.rarediseases.org.

State Children's Health Insurance Program (SCHIP). www.cms.gov/home/chip.asp.

Supplemental Security Income (SSI), Social Security Administration. www.ssa.gov/pubs/10026.html.

Glossary

504 Accommodation Plan: Planning document used in schools for children who require health-related services (including modified meals), but who are not enrolled in a special education program; mandated by the Rehabilitation Act of 1973.

achondroplasia: An inherited congenital disorder that is characterized by short stature, short limbs, normal trunk, and specific head/face features (large head, prominent forehead, low nasal bridge).

ADA. *See* Americans with Disabilities Act of 1990 (ADA).

Adequate Intake (AI): A recommended intake value based on observed or experimentally determined approximations or estimates of nutrient intake by a group (or groups) of healthy people that are assumed to be adequate; used when an RDA cannot be determined.

ADHD. *See* attention deficit hyperactivity disorder (ADHD).

ADL: Activities of daily living.

AGA: Appropriate for gestational age; includes consideration for degree of prematurity.

AI. *See* Adequate Intake (AI).

Americans with Disabilities Act of 1990 (ADA): Federal legislation enacted to protect persons with disabilities from discrimination.

anal stenosis: A condition in which the anus is narrowed.

anthropometric: Pertaining to the science of measuring the body, including height, length, weight, and the size of other body parts.

anticonvulsant: Medications used to prevent or control the occurrence or severity of seizures; medication-nutrient interactions can affect metabolism of vitamins D, B-6, B-12, folic acid, and carnitine.

apnea: Cessation of breathing for a time; a sign of respiratory distress of multifactorial etiology, including prematurity and feeding problems in children with special health care needs.

arm span: The distance between a child's extended right and left middle fingers, measured across the back; sometimes used to estimate height.

ASD. *See under* autism.

aspiration: The drawing or sucking in of foreign material into the lungs, including food, liquid, or stomach contents; clinically significant aspiration requires consideration of non-oral feeding and/or surgery to protect the airway.

ataxia: Imbalance or lack of coordination of voluntary and involuntary movements; seen in neurological disorders (eg, cerebral palsy).

athetoid/athetosis: Condition of ceaseless, involuntary muscle movements; a form of cerebral palsy; can result in increased energy needs.

attention deficit hyperactivity disorder (ADHD): A neurological disorder that results in excessive activity (hyperactivity), impulsivity, and difficulties with focusing attention.

autism: A type of pervasive developmental disorder (PDD) that includes communication problems, ritualistic behaviors, and inappropriate social interactions; part of autism spectrum disorder (ASD).

BMI. *See* body mass index.

body mass index (BMI): An indicator of weight and height proportionality used in nutrition screening (BMI in 85th to 95th percentile indicates overweight; BMI > 95th percentile indicates obesity; BMI < 5th percentile indicates underweight). BMI = weight (kg)/height (m)^2.

bolus: Term used in enteral nutrition support to indicate a feeding administered at one time, usually by gastrostomy or nasogastric tube.

BPD. *See* bronchopulmonary dysplasia (BPD).

bronchopulmonary dysplasia (BPD): A chronic lung disorder; most commonly seen in children born prematurely, with low birth weight, or requiring prolonged mechanical ventilation; nutritional consequences can include feeding difficulties, slow growth, and increased energy needs.

calipers: An instrument with two hinged jaws used for measuring the thickness or diameter of an object.

catch-up growth: Rate of growth that is faster than expected, seen when a child who has experienced stunted growth due to a nutritional insult receives adequate energy and protein.

CDC: Centers for Disease Control and Prevention.

cerebral palsy (CP): A nonprogressive motor nerve disorder of the central nervous system; results in muscle coordination difficulties; different parts of the body are affected: hemiplegia affects only the right or left side, diplegia primarily affects the legs, and quadriplegia affects the whole body; movements may be described as spastic (increased tone) or dystonia (slow, rhythmic, twisting), athetoid (involuntary writhing movements), or ataxic (unbalanced jerky movements).

CF. *See* cystic fibrosis.

CHAMPUS. *See* TRICARE.

Children with Special Health Care Needs (CSHCN) program: Federal- (Title V) and state-funded program located in state health departments; promotes and coordinates services for children who have serious physical, behavioral, or emotional conditions that require health and related services beyond those generally required by children.

chronic lung disease of infancy (CLD): A suggested term to describe infants who continue to have a significant pulmonary dysfunction at 36 weeks gestational age.

chronic renal failure (CRF): Less than 25% renal function; may be due to congenital anatomical defects, inherited disease, untreated kidney infections, physical trauma or exposure to nephrotoxic chemicals.

chronic renal insufficiency (CRI): Less than 50% renal function; a progressive disorder that can lead to chronic renal failure.

cleft lip and cleft palate: Conditions occurring when tissues that usually form the lip or the roof of the mouth fail to grow together, creating a gap in the lip or a hole in the roof of the mouth; may be an isolated condition or may be associated with other syndromes; the cleft lip is usually repaired at approximately 3 months of age; the cleft palate is usually repaired at approximately 1 year of age.

CNS: Central nervous system.

congenital heart disease: A cardiac problem that is present at birth, involving one or more defects in the heart, the heart's valves, the veins leading to the heart or the connections among these various parts of the body; usually repaired by surgery early in life.

contracture: Static muscle shortening resulting from tonic spasm or fibrosis; frequently seen in individuals with cerebral palsy.

Cornelia de Lange: A genetic disorder that can lead to severe developmental anomalies.

corrected age: Age from birth, corrected for prematurity; 40 weeks minus gestational age at birth (eg, an infant born at 30 weeks' gestation has a corrected age of 2 weeks at 12 weeks after birth).

CP. *See* cerebral palsy.

crown-rump length: Length between a child's head and buttocks; sometimes used as an estimator of length.

CSHCN: Children with special health care needs. *See also* Children with Special Health Care Needs (CSHCN) program.

cystic fibrosis (CF): An inherited disorder of the endocrine glands, primarily the pancreas, pulmonary system, and sweat glands, characterized by abnormally thick luminal secretions.

diaphragmatic hernia: Protrusion of part of the stomach upwards through an abnormal opening between the thoracic and abdominal cavities; associated with respiratory, cardiac, and gastrointestinal problems.

Dietary Reference Intakes (DRIs): Generic term for a set of nutrient reference values; includes Estimated Average Requirement (EAR), Recommended Dietary Allowance (RDA), Adequate Intake (AI), Tolerable Upper Intake Level (UL), and Estimated Energy Requirement (EER).

Down syndrome: Trisomy 21; a genetic disorder in which the individual has an extra 21st chromosome; characterized by short stature, low muscle tone, cardiac and gastrointestinal problems, cognitive delay, and distinct facial appearance.

DRI. *See* Dietary Reference Intakes (DRIs).

dysphagia: Difficulty in swallowing.

EAR. *See* Estimated Average Requirement (EAR).

Early Head Start: Expansion of the Head Start program to serve low-income pregnant women, infants, and children to age 3 years; program components include education; social services; meals and snacks; health, nutrition, and dental screening and education.

early intervention services: Community-based, comprehensive therapeutic and educational services for infants and children up to 3 years of age with developmental delays; established by Part H of the federal Individuals With Disabilities Education Act (IDEA) of 1986 (now Part C of IDEA, 1997).

Early Periodic Screening, Diagnosis, and Treatment (EPSDT): Program within Medicaid for people younger than 22 years of age; provides medical and dental services; can often provide nutrition-related specialty services, depending on state restrictions.

EER. *See* Estimated Energy Requirement (EER).

encopresis: Fecal incontinence not due to organic defect or illness.

EPSDT. *See* Early Periodic Screening, Diagnosis, and Treatment (EPSDT).

Estimated Average Requirement (EAR): A daily nutrient intake value that is estimated to meet the requirement for half of the healthy individuals in a life state and gender group.

Estimated Energy Requirement (EER): DRI for energy; calculated using PAL.

failure to thrive: Refers to slowed rate of growth, usually describes weight loss, decreased rate of weight gain and/or decreased linear growth; also called undernutrition, delayed growth, growth faltering, and failure to grow.

fragile X: The most common cause of inherited mental impairment.

fundoplication: Surgical procedure that involves mobilizing the lower end of the esophagus and wrapping the fundus of the stomach around it; indicated by diminished function of lower esophageal sphincter or severe/chronic gastroesophageal reflux disease (GERD); sometimes done when placing a gastrostomy tube.

gag reflex: A normal reflex triggered by touching the soft palate or back of the throat, which raises the palate, retracts the tongue, and contracts the throat muscles; protects the airway from a bolus of food or liquid.

galactagogue: Substance that is ingested (foods, herbs, medications, etc), which has the effect of increasing breastmilk supply (induces lactation).

gastroesophageal reflux disease (GERD): Regurgitation of stomach contents upward through the lower esophageal sphincter into the esophagus, where they can be aspirated; results in uncomfortable, burning sensation; common cause of feeding and eating problems in infants and children with neuromuscular disabilities.

gastroschisis: A birth defect of incomplete closure of the abdominal wall.

gastrostomy tube: A feeding tube surgically placed through an opening from the abdomen to the stomach; tubes can also be placed endoscopically.

GERD. *See* gastroesophageal reflux disease (GERD).

GI: Gastrointestinal.

glycogen storage diseases: Caused by deficiencies of enzymes that regulate the synthesis or degradation of glycogen; hypoglycemia can be life-threatening; treatment can include nocturnal drip feedings of a carbohydrate-containing solution, or raw cornstarch therapy.

granulation tissue: Connective tissue that forms on the surface of a wound, ulcer, or inflamed tissue surface.

Head Start: Federally funded preschool program for children ages 3 to 5 years from low-income families; includes children with special needs; program components include parent education, meals and snacks, health, nutrition, and dental screening, and education.

health maintenance organization (HMO): A type of managed care.

height-age equivalent: Age at which current length or height would fall at the 50th percentile on the length-for-age or height-for-age growth chart.

Hirschsprung's disease: Congenital absence of nerves in the smooth muscle wall of the colon, resulting in buildup of feces and widening of the bowel (megacolon).

HMO. *See* health maintenance organization (HMO).

hydrocephalus: A congenital or acquired condition with accumulation of cerebrospinal fluid within the skull; characterized by enlarged head, prominent forehead, mental deterioration, and seizures.

hypersensitivity: Abnormal sensitivity; exaggerated response by the body to a stimulus, such as touch, taste, or smell; in feeding problems, hypersensitivity includes adverse reaction or refusal to have mouth touched or teeth brushed, gagging or negative reaction to food in mouth, and tactile defensiveness.

hypertonia: Increased muscle tone; facial hypertonia may result in oral-motor feeding difficulties such as bite reflexes and retracted upper lip.

hypotonia: Diminished muscle tone; can result in poor suck and feeding difficulties.

IBW. *See* ideal body weight (IBW).

ICC. *See* Interagency Coordinating Council (ICC).

IDEA. *See* Individual with Disabilities Education Act of 1997 (IDEA).

ideal body weight (IBW): Weight at 50th percentile for current age.

IEP. *See* Individualized Education Program (IEP).

IFSP. *See* Individualized Family Service Plan (IFSP).

Indian Health Services: Federal program to provide health services to Native Americans.

Individualized Education Program (IEP): Planning document required annually for special education services in public schools serving children older than 3 years; outlines specific goals, activities, and timelines.

Individualized Family Service Plan (IFSP): Planning document required for services for children from birth to 3 years of age enrolled in early intervention services; includes specific goals, activities, and timelines.

Individual with Disabilities Education Act of 1997 (IDEA): Federal education legislation; Part C includes early intervention services.

Interagency Coordinating Council (ICC): Each state providing early intervention services under IDEA (Part C) has an ICC located in the state government.

IVH: Intraventricular hemorrhage; graded 1 (mild) to 4 (major); in premature infants, may be associated with subsequent neurological damage and developmental disability.

jaw grading: Ability to control the degree of movement of the lower jaw; a feeding skill important in accepting food from a spoon and in biting and chewing.

jaw retraction: Involuntary movement of the jaw backward, making it difficult to open the mouth voluntarily; a common oral-motor feeding problem that interferes with the ability to handle food textures.

low birth weight (LBW): Used to describe a newborn weighing less than 2,500 g (5.5 lb) and less than 38 weeks' gestation.

macrocephaly: Excessively large size of head.

Marfan syndrome: Congenital disorder of the connective tissue characterized by excessive length of the fingers and toes and other deformities.

MCT. *See* medium-chain triglycerides (MCT).

Medicaid: Federal medical assistance program for children from low-income families; often matched by state funds.

medium-chain triglycerides (MCT): Triglycerides with eight to ten carbon atoms. MCTs do not require bile for digestion and are usually easily digested.

microcephaly: Small head size in relation to age and other growth parameters; may reflect inadequate brain growth; common feature of neurological damage before or immediately after birth.

modified barium swallow: A radiologic study of the oral and pharyngeal cavities to evaluate the swallowing mechanism; foods and liquids are mixed with barium and the feeding is recorded on videotape; also called *videofluoroscopic swallowing study* (VFSS).

munching: Oral-motor feeding developmental stage characterized by up-and-down movement of the jaw; occurs before development of rotary chewing.

myelomeningocele. *See* spina bifida.

myotonic dystrophy: An inherited autosomal dominant neuromuscular disorder that occurs in adults; characterized by progressive muscle weakness, wasting, and mytonia.

nasogastric feeding: A form of enteral nutrition support; tube runs from nose into stomach; usually used temporarily (eg, less than 3 months).

National School Breakfast and Lunch Program: School program in which children receive a balanced morning and midday meal; sponsored by the USDA's Child Nutrition Program.

necrotizing enterocolitis: A sudden inflammatory bowel disorder that occurs primarily in premature or LBW infants; causes blood to move away from the gastrointestinal tract, resulting in necrosis with bacterial invasion of the intestinal wall.

Nellhaus chart: Standard reference for head circumference in infants and children from birth to age 18 years.

NICU: Neonatal intensive care unit.

Noonan syndrome: A disorder marked by short stature, webbing of the neck, mental retardation, and craniofacial features (wide mouth, protruding upper lip).

obstipation: Constipation resulting in accumulation of feces with development of colon distention; leads to fecal impaction.

obstructive lesions: Conditions where a normal body passage is partly or completely obstructed; examples of those affecting eating and nutrition include pyloric stenosis, tracheoesophageal fistula, duodenal atresia.

oral rehydration therapy (ORT): Slow oral administration of glucose, sodium, potassium, and chloride to replace fluid and electrolyte losses and correct extracellular fluid volume after mild or severe dehydration.

ORT. *See* oral rehydration therapy (ORT).

PAL. *See* physical activity level (PAL).

palmar grasp: Hand movement in which the palm rather than the fingertips make contact with an object for grasping; developmental stage that is an important precursor to self-feeding.

PDD: Pervasive developmental disorder.

phasic bite reflex: Opening and closing of the jaw that occurs when the gums and teeth are stimulated.

phenylketonuria (PKU): An amino acid disorder inherited as an autosomal recessive; marked by the deficiency of the enzyme that converts phenylalanine to tyrosine; accumulation of phenylalanine in the blood can lead to mental retardation and other neurological problems; identified in newborn screening; treatment includes a special diet with medical foods.

physical activity level (PAL): Coefficient used to determine estimated energy requirements (EER).

Pierre-Robin syndrome: Disorder characterized by small lower jaw and abnormal smallness of the tongue; often with cleft palate or with other malformations; results in respiratory and feeding problems; also called *Robin sequence*.

pincer grasp: Refined, mature hand movement in which the thumb and index finger are used to grasp a small object; a developmental stage that is an important skill in self-feeding.

PKU. *See* phenylketonuria (PKU).

positioning: Physical management of posture and body alignment to support daily living skills such as standing and eating.

post-ictal: Following a seizure.

Prader-Willi syndrome: Genetic disorder of chromosome 15 marked by hypotonia, short stature, hyperphagia, and developmental disabilities; characterized by poor feeding in infancy, and when not carefully managed, excessive weight gain in children and adults.

preterm: Term used to describe an infant who is born prematurely at less than 38 weeks' gestation.

RDA. *See* Recommended Dietary Allowance (RDA).

recognized medical authority: Term in federal regulations pertaining to Child Nutrition Programs that refers to a physician, physician's assistant, registered nurse, nurse practitioner, registered dietitian, or other specialist identified by the state agency (eg, Department of Education).

Recommended Dietary Allowance (RDA): The intake that meets the nutrient need of almost all (97%–98%) of individuals in a group.

Rett syndrome: A neurological disorder of females, marked by progressive neurological deterioration, seizures, and cognitive impairment.

Robin sequence. *See* Pierre-Robin syndrome.

rooting reflex: Newborn reflex in which the infant turns his head toward the hand or nipple stroking his cheek, and initiates sucking.

rotary chewing: Movement of jaw side-to-side and up-and-down to grind and mash food; a mature developmental feeding stage in which a wide variety of food textures can be handled.

Rubinstein-Taybi syndrome: A specific pattern of physical features and developmental disabilities that occur together in a consistent fashion. Individuals with Rubinstein-Taybi syndrome have short stature, developmental delay, similar facial features, and broad thumbs and first toes.

SCHIP. *See* State Children's Health Insurance Program (SCHIP).

scoliosis: Lateral curvature of the vertebral column; associated with some congenital and neurological disorders.

seizure disorder: Involuntary movement or changes in consciousness or behavior brought on by abnormal bursts of electrical activity in the brain; seizures can be classified as general or partial; when seizures occur repeatedly they are diagnosed as epilepsy.

sensory integration (SI) therapy: Techniques, used by some speech-language therapists, occupational therapists, or physical therapists, aimed at helping children sort out and organize their senses, thereby improving hypersensitivities or hyposensitivities and fine-motor skills.

SGA. *See* small for gestational age (SGA).

sickle cell: An autosomal recessive genetic, blood disorder, with overdominance, characterized by red blood cells that assume an abnormal, rigid, sickle shape.

SI therapy. *See* sensory integration (SI) therapy.

sitting height: Length between a child's head and buttocks; sometimes used as an estimator of height.

skeletal dysplasia: A group of congenital abnormalities of the bone and cartilage that are characterized by short stature.

small for gestational age (SGA): Birth weight less than 10th percentile for age.

spastic: Increased muscle tone and stiffness; descriptor for cerebral palsy.

Special Olympics: An international program of year-round sports training and athletic competition for children and adults with mental retardation.

Special Supplemental Nutrition Program for Women, Infants, and Children (WIC): A federal program providing foods, infant formula, and nutrition education to pregnant and breastfeeding women, infants, and children younger than 5 years of age.

spina bifida: A congenital defect in which part of the spinal column fails to close completely during fetal development, resulting in a hernia (containing the spinal cord, the meninges, and cerebral spinal fluid) along the spinal column; higher lesions result in greater limitations in mobility; long-term nutritional risks include overweight, constipation, and reduced energy needs; also called *myelomeningocele*.

SSI. *See* Supplemental Security Income (SSI).

State Children's Health Insurance Program (SCHIP): A federal Medicaid children's health insurance program created in 1997; optional program for states to offer uninsured or underinsured children who generally do not qualify for Medicaid; different names in different states.

static encephalopathy: A general term for a neurological or brain disorder that is stable.

steatorrhea: Excessive amounts of fats in the feces; stool characterized by light color and offensive odor; feces float.

sucking: A more mature up-and-down movement of the tongue and jaw, with negative pressure, to extract liquid from a nipple.

suckling: The earliest intake pattern in infants; the lower jaw and tongue elevate and move back and forth, using pressure on the nipple to extract fluid during feeding; replaced by sucking.

Supplemental Security Income (SSI): Federal- and state-funded program that provides supplemental income to offset expenses for children with disabilities who come from low-income families.

TEE. *See* Total Energy Expenditure.

texture: Consistency of food at the time it is served; generally based on amount of mastication required before swallowing.

Tolerable Upper Intake Level (UL): The maximum level of daily nutrient intake that is likely to pose no risk of adverse effects for almost all individuals in the general population; unless otherwise specified, the UL represents total intake from food, water, and supplements; ULs are not established for vitamin K, riboflavin, vitamin B-12, pantothenic acid, biotin, or carotenoids.

tongue lateralization: Ability to move the tongue voluntarily from side to side from its midline position; developmental stage in feeding that signals the ability to manipulate food inside the mouth.

tongue retraction: Involuntary tongue movement toward the back of the mouth on presentation of food, spoon, or cup; blocks the normal steps to swallowing.

tongue thrust: Forceful protrusion of the tongue, often in response to an oral stimulus, such as a spoon or food; interferes with moving food from the front of the mouth to the back for swallowing.

tonic bite reflex: Involuntary bite reflex with associated tension; the bite is not easily released (eg, appears that child is biting spoon or finger and cannot release it).

Total Energy Expenditure (TEE): The intake that meets the average energy expenditure of individuals at the reference height, weight, and age.

tracheomalacia: Softening of the cartilage rings in the trachea; results in feeding difficulties with risk of apnea and aspiration during eating.

transpyloric feeding: Nutrition support in which a tube extends from the nose through the stomach, past the pyloric valve, into the first part of the small intestine; used primarily when the person is at risk for aspiration of stomach contents.

TRICARE: A health insurance program for families in the US military; formerly called CHAMPUS.

triceps skinfold measure: Measurement of the skin and subcutaneous fat layer around the triceps muscle; used with arm circumference measurement to estimate fat and muscle stores.

trisomy 13: A genetic disorder where there are three copies of chromosome 13 that result in a syndrome characterized by mental retardation and defects to the central nervous system and heart. (also known as Patau syndrome)

trisomy 18: A genetic disorder where there are 3 copies of chromosome 18 and characterized by developmental issues and medical complications that are more potentially life-threatening in the early months and years of life.

trisomy 21. *See* Down syndrome.

Turner syndrome: Disorder in females from the absence of one X chromosome; marked by short stature, ovarian failure, and cardiac problems.

UL. *See* Tolerable Upper Intake Level (UL).

ventricular septal defect (VSD): Cardiac anomaly that requires medical or surgical treatment; usually requires increased energy needs.

very low birth weight (VLBW): Descriptor of a premature infant who weighs less than 1,500 g (3.5 1b) at birth.

VFSS. *See* videofluoroscopic swallowing study (VFSS).

videofluoroscopic swallowing study (VFSS): A radiologic study of the oral and pharyngeal cavities to evaluate the swallowing mechanism; foods and liquids are mixed with barium and the feeding is recorded on videotape; also called *modified barium swallow study.*

VLBW. *See* very-low-birth-weight (VLBW).

VSD. *See* ventricular septal defect (VSD).

weight-age equivalent: Age at which current weight would fall at the 50th percentile on the weight-for-age growth chart.

WHO. World Health Organization.

WIC. *See* Special Supplemental Nutrition Program for Women, Infants, and Children (WIC).

Williams syndrome: A disorder characterized by distinctive facial features (large lips, small eyes, depressed nasal bridge), growth and developmental delays, cardiac defects, and possible hypercalcemia in infancy.

z score: A z score reflects how many standard deviations above or below the population mean a raw score is. For instance, on a scale that has a mean of 500 and a standard deviation of 100, a score of 450 would equal a z score of $(450-500)/100 = -50/100 = -0.50$, which indicates that the score is half a standard deviation below the mean.

Index

Page number followed by *b* signifies box; *f*, figure; *t*, table.